Diary of a Sex Fiend

Girl with a One Track Mind

Diary of a Sex Fiend

Girl with a One Track Mind

Abby Lee

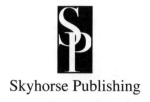

Skyhorse Publishing

First Skyhorse Publishing Edition Copyright © 2007

Originally published by Ebury Press, The Random House Group, Ltd.

www.skyhorsepublishing.com

10 9 8 7 6 5 4 3 2 1

Library of Congress Cataloging-in-Publication Data

Lee, Abby.
  Diary of a sex fiend : girl with a one-track mind / Abby Lee.
     p. cm.
  Reprint, originally published as: Girl with a one track mind. London :
Ebury Publishing, 2006.
  ISBN-13: 978-1-60239-015-7 (pbk. : alk. paper)
  ISBN-10: 1-60239-015-0 (pbk. : alk. paper)
  1. Women--Sexual behavior--Case studies. 2. Man-woman relationships-
-Case studies. I. Lee Abby. Girl with a one track mind. II. Title.

HQ29.L388 2007
306.7082'0942--dc22

                                                    2006039359

Printed in Canada

Acknowledgements

There are a few people I would like to show my appreciation to, for without them, this book would not have been possible.

Thank you to Jake Lingwood, Rachel Rayner and the rest of the team at Ebury Press for their encouragement and passion for the book.

Thank you to my agent Simon Benham, who 'got it' from day one.

Thank you to Ian Vince, for the introduction and helpful advice.

Thank you to David Bloom, for the guidance and support.

Thank you to Alex Marsh, the writer of JonnyB's Private Secret Diary, who has been a trusted friend as well as a brilliant sounding board.

Thank you to my parents, who have been wonderful, supportive and loving. And who I hope never read the book.

Finally, I must say a huge thanks to all the readers of my blog. Their positive feedback played a part in my writing this and I am grateful for all their support over the last two years.

Abby Lee is 32, lives in London and works in the film industry.

Her website detailing her real-life sex diaries has had over 2 million visitors and now attracts more than 100,000 readers every month. It was recently awarded Best British or Irish Blog at the 2006 Bloggies.

You can read her blog at:
www.girlwithaonetrackmind.blogspot.com

Does thinking about sex all the time mean there's something wrong with me?

It's a question I ask myself on an hourly basis. Surely not every woman thinks about shagging constantly? Is it common for other women to look at men's crotches as they walk down the street? Do most women weigh up the fuckability of every man they meet?

I just don't know – I wish I did. I'm beginning to worry that I might be some kind of freak; that because I have a one-track mind it might make me different to other women.

I know that most people don't have a problem with talking casually about sex. My own friends appear quite happy to sit in a pub, swapping *Sex and the City* anecdotes and joking about rabbit vibrators. But, the thing is, if I get into more detail and mention something like, say, wanting to try out a cock ring on a guy while fingering his arse, they all suddenly become rather quiet or jump up and volunteer to buy the next round. And I'd be left sitting there staring at the bartender's trouser bulge, worrying that yet again I had embarrassed myself with my sordid fixation.

I guess I've always suspected I might be a little different. Back when we were in our twenties my female friends would happily chat about dieting, make-up techniques and how to flirt with a man, but I wasn't interested in all that. I was more focussed on becoming a successful camera assistant in the movie industry, and busily trying to figure out if anal sex would hurt and whether the missionary position would give me enough orgasms to be fully satisfied. (It did, and it definitely does.)

I thought that maybe it was just an age thing then, and that by the time we were all in our thirties my friends' sex drives would match my own adventurous streak. But now that we're thirty something most of my friends are either married with kids in tow, or else they want to be and are desperately trying to find a life partner by any means necessary.

So I suppose I do sometimes feel like I have to keep up a façade when I'm with my mates; it frustrates me that I have to hide what is in my head, to spare me or them from getting embarrassed. I wish I could just be myself and talk openly with them, but how can I be truthful and tell them I want to try out group sex when they only seem to care about finding that *one* special man to have sex with?

But even if I'm the odd one out I'm still sure there's plenty of fun to be had besides the quest for Mr Right. Why search for a knight in shining armour when you can have a great ride with just a few vodka-based cocktails and a cheap sex toy to hand? When you're 32, single and horny, why not have some fun?

With all these thoughts going round my head, I decided to keep a diary. It seemed like the best way to express all my anxieties, neuroses and needs without any risk to my friendships. I reckoned that writing everything down would be the only way I could be truly open about sex; I could talk about my sexuality and desires as a woman and not have to worry or care what people might think, and whether they'd judge me or not. It would be liberating.

I also realised that if I had a record of everything that happened and how I'd felt about it, I'd be able to look back over all the sordid/tragic/glorious aspects of my sex life and laugh or cry about it later. I could be objective about it, and maybe I'd finally be able to work out why I was so preoccupied with sex. Perhaps I could even *do* something about it as a result.

So for the past year I have faithfully kept this diary. In order to write with complete truth and openness, I've done it anonymously: I haven't told my friends, family or anyone at work about it. I have written it free from the judgment or the opinions of others, but I really hope that nobody I know ever reads it. I'm not ashamed about any of the things I have done, but I don't really want my nearest and dearest to know how obsessed I am about sex, let alone the people I have to work with in a professional capacity.

To protect my anonymity and others' right to privacy I have refrained from divulging too much personal information and have changed minor details like names, locations and dates, but all the characters, their dialogue and the events that occurred are real. These have been recounted as accurately as possible (give or take one or two Martinis).

1

January

Quite frankly I need a shag.

The last person I slept with was my ex, Steven, and that was months ago. Now I'm gagging for some more action.

Last night I thought I'd struck it lucky. The whole of London was partying. It seemed like I was surrounded by possibilities; everywhere I looked, there were men with potential. So when I encountered not one, not two, but three promising blokes, I figured something would happen with one of them, right?

With some friends from work egging me on, and the help of a few beers, I plucked up the courage to approach one of the guys. I'll call him Party Boy.

As we chatted he seemed funny, sweet and kind. I felt confident enough to flirt a little and even blurted out that he had a nice arse, but he said he didn't want to 'take things any further' and left me standing there on my own by the bar. Result: *confused*.

Round two: Brainy Bloke.

Shy, but witty and clever. We got into a deep conversation about ID cards. I thought I was in there with a chance, but midway through my polemic on the Labour Party's authoritarianism, he walked off to chat to a pretty blonde girl instead. Result: *annoyed*.

Round three: Tall Man.

Smart, and handsome in a cute way. After leaving the club, we drunkenly kissed in the street, then suddenly he said he had to go home to get some sleep and left me there waiting for a night bus. Result: *gutted*.

I can't understand what went so wrong. I think I'm not a bad looker (if you're into curvy brunettes who go for a run three times a week); I reckon I'm reasonably intelligent, perhaps even funny. I know I'm clumsy and have big feet, but surely having big boobs balances out the negatives?

Something must be really unappealing about me or my approach; I thought at least *one* of these blokes would result in some action. I was wrong – on three counts. To misread *all three* situations so badly must surely mean I've lost my mojo? If so, how do I get it back?

And why is this happening now, when I'm in my sexual prime?

I suppose doing a Bridget Jones and sitting in on a Saturday night wondering where all the good men are, doesn't help matters. But after three rejections, I'm not quite sure if I can pluck up my courage and try a new approach just yet. I need a little time to recover.

I'm going to have to do something soon though, because my vibrators are getting a hell of a bashing.

Monday 3rd January

Combine horniness with a new broadband connection and you get a girl who is spending far, far too long on-line.

It's all getting too much for me; the fast downloading speed has meant I keep looking at porn, and then I end up yet again with my hands in my nether regions. What a timewaster I am.

It's not just the porn-surfing either. I've discovered weblogs too, and find them totally compelling. I love finding out what goes on in other people's lives, especially the ones who have more, and more interesting, sex than me. I'm starting to get addicted to some of them and check them every day for new posts.

Not all of my favourites are erotic – well, obviously erotic. Some of them are very funny, and if there's one thing I like – other than good sex – it's someone with a killer sense of humour. If they can make me laugh there's nothing like that endorphin rush; it's a fantastic release of energy, just like a good orgasm. And I certainly like those.

That's probably why a man with a good sense of humour has always made more of an impression on me than someone with a handsome face or who is skilled in bed. It's a very sexy quality for a man to have; when he makes me laugh, I loosen up and then I begin to feel at ease, and *then* it starts to turn me on.

So I can't read the weblogs which make me giggle the most without wondering about the men who write them. They make me feel so good that I find myself wanting to know what they're like in real life, and if they know what pleasure they give me when they write. And that they turn me on. I doubt it.

There's one which stands out. This guy – I'll call him Blog Boy – has me in fits of laughter with every post. I love his style – it's not just that it's hilarious, it's also very honest, and that makes me curious about just how warm and genuine he might be in real life. And yes, he makes my pants wet when I read him, even though I have no idea what he looks like or if he's single.

That sense of humour alone was enough to make me take the plunge and email him to see if he fancied a beer. It's probably stupid – he could be a weird internet psycho for all I know, but I still have to know what might happen if we meet up. If he's anything like his on-line persona it could be *very* interesting. You never know what might be on the cards. If I get my wicked way with him, that is.

Thursday 6th January

When I tell people what I do for a living, they tend to get all excited and start asking me questions like:

'Ooh! Do you meet lots of famous people, then? Who's the most famous actor you have worked with?'

I wearily mention that being a camera assistant in the film industry often means having to be at work at 5 a.m. and then getting home after 10 p.m., and that the constant tiredness rather takes the glitz and the glamour off being surrounded by celebrities.

Because I am freelance, it means I also have to be ready to work at all times – with no preparation – because a job could come up at the last minute. The last minute being, for example, 6 a.m. this morning.

Last night I stumbled in drunk from a gig at about 2 a.m. and fell into bed, only to be woken by the phone a few hours later.

What cock-sucking-bastard-wanker is phoning me at this fucking hour? I thought, as I tried to recall whether I gave my number out last night and wished the painful pounding in my head would go away.

The call went to voicemail, and a moment later, I picked up my mobile to listen to the message, just in case.

It was an emergency plea. Film freelancers get a lot of these. Invariably they need you *now* because their regular person is ill/hungover/been sacked/gone onto another (better) project, and they've got work for you, but *can you be there in an hour?* That sort of thing.

I had to think it over: I felt rotten. Hardly any sleep, my head like a fucking vice, the knowledge that if I said yes I would have to be on my feet for more than 12 hours – none of this was appealing.

Then again there's not much work just now and I have tons of bills to pay, so I ended up calling them back and saying I'd be there as soon as I could. Like a doctor grabbing their medical kit, I did a last-minute check on the work bag I always have standing by to make sure I had everything:

★ Comfortable boots – check. [Must be waterproof, warm and not give you blisters after wearing them for 17+ hours]
★ Comfortable trousers with many pockets – check. [You can never have too many pockets as a camera assistant]
★ 'Coolmax' socks – check. [To soak up the (inevitable large amounts of) sweat that your feet will produce during the day]
★ Non-cotton t-shirt – check [Ditto on the sweat. Plus, having an ironic slogan on your chest always brightens people's days and prevents boredom on set]

★ Super-duper fleece – check. [It's a prerequisite that all crew members wear a fleece with the insignia of the last film they worked on – preferably a major movie. That way, people know you are in demand, and not some small fry who only works in TV]

★ Thermal leggings + vest – check. [Just in case. You never know when you'll be standing outside for 15 hours freezing your tits off]

★ Second pair of socks – check. [In case of leakage, or if your toes just get damn cold]

★ Waterproof trousers – check. [Nothing like working in wet jeans, yuck]

★ Waterproof jacket/coat – check. [Must be water*proof*, not water-*repellent*. There IS a difference]

★ Scarf + gloves– check.

★ Warm hat – check. [If it's waterproof too, even better]

★ Work belt – check. [Must be able to carry the weight of heavy-duty tools]

★ Work bag for the belt – check. [For all my worldly goods and the camera paraphernalia]

★ Radio-holster – check. [For the annoyingly heavy walkie-talkies]

★ Covert ear-piece – check. [So we can receive/give instructions quietly on set]

★ Pink see-through lacy thong with a sequinned heart on the front panel – check. [OK, not a necessity, but after all the 'manly' heavy work-wear I have to don, I like to feel sexy and feminine underneath it all]

Aside from the last-minute bookings, there is one thing, one *major* thing that I do dislike about working in film: being knackered all the time is not conducive to my regular frigs.

When faced with four hours' sleep or three hours 45 minutes' sleep between work, I choose the sleep almost every time. Sometimes a girl is just too tired to have a rub.

Sunday 9th January

Blog Boy has returned my email! And, I am happy to say, is flirting back with me on-line. More importantly, he has agreed to meet me for a drink next week, and I'm overjoyed.

There is *something* about the way this guy writes that I find utterly captivating; I have to get to know him. I probably shouldn't get my hopes too high but I can't help being excited about seeing him in the flesh.

I can't help but wonder what he looks like naked.

Tuesday 11th January

Although I got a result from contacting Blog Boy, it's clear I still need to perfect my chat-up skills because I just missed a fantastic opportunity because I wasn't confident enough.

There I was this evening, having a relaxed glass of wine in a pub with my old college friend Fiona, and who should walk in but my number one crush of the moment: Graham Coxon. All I could do was throw shy glances towards the guy who was the guitarist in Blur. I had no idea how to approach him though. I went through the options in my head:

★ The sycophantic route?
  'Hi Graham, I think you're amazingly talented, you are a true spokesman for our time.'

★ The empathetic route?
'Hi Graham, I truly feel your angst. Your lyrics have really touched me.'

★ The name-dropping route?
'Hi Graham, I'm Abby. I used to work with Kevin at EMI; you know him?'

★ The blagging route?
'Hi Graham, I work in film. Ever thought of acting? I could put you in touch with the right people.'

★ The egotistical route?
'Hi Graham, I think you're great. I'd love to shoot your next video. Here's my card.'

★ The chat-up route?
'Hi there. I just had to come over and say hi – you have lovely eyes, you know. Can I buy you a beer?'

★ The totally unrealistic, yet I can always dream route?
'Hi Graham. I think you're a superb guitarist, but I'm not sure who would win in a contest between yourself and Justin Hawkins from The Darkness. Perhaps you should bring him over to my place and then I'll be able to decide which of you is the most skilled musician.

'Of course it's not *obligatory* that you are naked whilst you play, but it will give you extra points and assist me with my decision. The winner of the contest gets to shag me; the runner-up, wins a blow job. If it's a tie, you'll just have to simultaneously share me, I'm afraid. Best of luck!'

Obviously I did none of the above. After finishing my wine and saying goodbye to Fiona, the only bit of Graham I got close to was his voice, on high volume on my iPod. Oh well, I can but dream.

Wednesday 12th January

This desire for sex … it's starting to interfere with work. It's getting harder to focus when I keep checking out my colleagues' arses. I should be concentrating on cleaning camera lenses but I'm getting distracted by the thought of cock, and if I drop such an expensive piece of equipment, no one will want to hire me.

But films crews are largely male, so I'm surrounded by men all day and this is playing hell with my current sexual frustration. I'm beginning to fantasise about shagging some of them. It's not good; you can't mix business and pleasure. I'm the only woman in my department and I want to be taken seriously on the film floor.

Still, I'm bored of having no action and there's so much out there to tempt me. Surely being single means I should be having lots of fun?

Friday 14th January

Finally I got a chance to perfect my flirting skills; last night I met up with Blog Boy.

God, was he handsome. Well over six feet tall, dirty blond hair and a huge grin to match the sparkle in his bright blue eyes. Yum. As I'd expected, and hoped, he was every bit as smart and warm as he'd come across in the blog; I found myself laughing out loud at his jokes. When he went to the loo I couldn't stop myself having a good look at his arse too. Very nice.

Five hours zipped past and I was completely relaxed and enjoying myself no end. I was doing well – even though we'd talked non-stop and got through plenty of booze I'd managed not to mention sex once. I was worried he'd be able to tell that all that was running through my head was hardcore porn images of me and him fucking, but I don't think he caught on, thank God.

With some regret we had to end things at midnight because I had to get up for work at 5 a.m. today. It was so annoying; I just wanted to know if he was as attracted to me as I was to him, and if he wanted to see me again, but as luck would have it, as he walked me to my bus stop our arms kept touching and that made us both giggle self-consciously. I held my breath, hoping we might snog before my bus pulled up.

As if he'd read my mind, Blog Boy leaned in to kiss me and gently rested his hand on my back. I had my answer. I finally knew the attraction was mutual: we snogged for over half an hour. Sod the bus.

He got me so heated up I found it very difficult to just leave him there – I could feel his erection pressing against his jeans – and I wanted him so badly. But I had to go so that I could get some sleep before work today. Happily, we arranged to meet up again next week – just before I go away to New York on holiday, and yes, as I sat on the bus I had a big smile all over my face, and sopping wet knickers. I didn't sleep much for thinking about him, which was a bit inconvenient after a 15-hour day on the set.

If he's as good in the flesh as he was in my fantasy, I think we'll be having some fun together.

Saturday 15th January

I can't stop thinking about Blog Boy; it's like being a school girl again, and that's making me feel all nostalgic. It reminds me of my first boyfriend Danny and what a huge crush I had on him too.

I was 16 and naïve. Danny was tall and good-looking with dark brown hair, intense green eyes and a gruff voice. We were in English class together. The first day I saw him I *knew*. I said to my friend Kathy, 'This is the guy I am going to lose my virginity with.'

And I just *knew* I would. And that he would be mine. It wasn't that I was super-confident about obtaining hot men, just that I had a feeling somewhere in my solar plexus that this boy and I were *meant* for each other.

Within two months, we were together.

We used to bunk off class to be with each other and hang out in the park, me smoking, him smiling. And we would kiss these innocent kisses – not like now, when I get all hot and bothered and have to adjust my clothes – but the ones where you look at each other and as your lips touch, you taste sweetness and feel a spark that is intoxicating and rejuvenating at the same time.

And we would fumble. He fumbled. I fumbled. We were fumblers; inexperienced, but in love, so whatever he did I enjoyed. I adored him. He worshipped me. And when *the time* came, he was the sweetest, gentlest person on the planet, thinking of everything.

Him: 'Do you have some towels?'
Me: 'Towels?'
Him: 'Yes, preferably dark ones.'

Me: 'Um, dark? Towels?'

Him *(whispering conspiratorially)*: 'You know, in case there's *blood* ...'

Me: 'BLOOD?'

Him: 'Um, yeah, you might bleed a little ...'

Me: 'I might bleed? What? No one said there'd be blood!'

Him *(trying to calm me)*: 'No, no, no. Just in case though, we don't want to mess your sheets up. I'll be careful; you probably won't bleed anyway ...'

I trusted him, so I went and got some towels and the condoms and we got ourselves ready.

Him: 'Now are you *sure* you want to do this? We don't have to, you know ...'

Me: 'It's now or never. Let's do it.'

And we did. Of course there was *no* blood, which, after that build-up, disappointed me somewhat; I felt that maybe it should have been more dramatic or something.

But it was OK; not bad, not terrible. I think we both enjoyed it, mostly, but neither of us was experienced. He had only had sex once before and at this point, I had no idea what an orgasm was, so the experience was enjoyable but nothing to write home about.

Not that we hadn't tried to make me climax. *Boy* we tried. We'd gone in search of my clitoris countless times, and some-times I'd be shouting:

'Yes! Yes! That's it!'

And him (coming up for air) saying:

'Sorry, where was that again?'

And, of course, then we couldn't find it, but since I didn't even know how to bring *myself* off at that point, there was no point expecting *him* to be able to get me there.

It wasn't until a few months after we broke up that I finally discovered the pleasure of self-pleasure, which was bad timing, but I've never looked back since.

Monday 17th January

Yet again I've been thinking about sex all day. I've been rushed off my feet for the best part of 14 hours at work, so there was no chance of taking a sneaky break to try to alleviate my horniness. It wasn't till I was driving home that I could finally slide my hand in between my legs and reach the part of me that had been aching to be touched all day.

Not that this was easy:

1) I had three layers of clothing to get through: waterproof insulated trousers, thermal leggings and a black lacy Lycra thong;
2) I had to steer the car on the motorway at 70 miles an hour with only one hand;
3) I was interrupted by calls and texts whilst I was driving/ playing and had to keep removing my hand to check my phone.

For almost an hour I was on the brink, but I couldn't risk orgasm-induced temporary blindness on a dual carriageway, so when I finally got home this evening, I bolted inside, kicked off my boots, dragged down my trousers and my thermals, and tugged down my pants.

And do you know what happened? For all my randiness the 5 a.m. starts, the long day and the sleep-deprivation finally got to me, and all I could manage was a bully wank.

This is where you've mildly got the horn but you're tired/had a long day/been wanking all day anyway and then you force yourself to masturbate on top of all that. Of course consent is involved, it's not like you have to coerce yourself into grabbing your own genitals – *oh come on, honey, you'll like it, I promise!* – more that you feel you *should* have a play, even given the state you're in, and you really try to enjoy yourself, but your heart's just not in it. Which may lead to:

a) not being able to climax
b) or it taking ages to climax
c) or a climax which is hardly worth it

In my exhaustion I ended up passing out, waking four hours later with my right hand still lying between my thighs and my clit still pulsing. I was robbed! How dare I? I'd been dying for this all day and I hadn't even had the decency to complete the task at hand. Outrageous!

So, with some determination, it has to be said, I dragged myself out of my slumber and *forced* myself to endure a few minutes of extreme pleasure.

This resulted in an orgasm that was far from spectacular, but still, it was delicious to imagine that it was Blog Boy's hand doing the business.

Tuesday 18th January

I'm not sure that this diary is helping me with my sex obsession. How else can I explain sending this text to my ex, Steven, earlier today?

'I want to taste you again. Lick and suck you deeply. I am so turned on thinking about your lovely cock in my mouth. Feel like something sweet to eat? I can be at yours in two hours.'

I sent this to the man that cheated on me with a younger woman; I must be crazy.

I quickly called Fiona to get some moral support and some sanity.

'Why the hell did you contact him again, Abby? After what he did to you, why lower yourself? He's just bad news; if you want sex that badly, find someone new!' she screamed at me down the phone.

I know she's right, but just the thought of some hot cock action stopped me thinking clearly. Thankfully, though, fate dealt me a good hand: Steven turned me down, saying that he had other plans.

So I am still frustrated but I'm very relieved that nothing happened: Steven is in my past for a good reason and I'd like him to stay that way.

Even if he was fantastic in the sack.

Wednesday 19th January

I just packed my thermals and waterproof clothing for a few days' work filming on location and I added a few extras:

★ 2 x see-through lacy pants (one black, one pink)
★ 1 x satin g-string (black)
★ 1 x French knickers (black with a cream trim)

I threw in an assortment of condoms (plain, ribbed and flavoured) too, so you could say that I have something other than work on my mind right now.

It's all Tony's fault. A new colleague of mine – with gorgeous eyes – he has been flirting with me all week. Our conversation is filled with sexual innuendo and it's got to the point where even the slightest joke seems like a blatant come-on.

What's a girl like me to do? I know that fucking someone from work is a really bad idea, but I can't help myself – I need a shag so badly! And being away from home all week and staying in the same hotel as Tony doesn't help matters.

It's no good. I think I am going to have to seize the next opportunity that arises – even if it is with someone from work.

I just wish it were Blog Boy instead, but I've got to wait for that until filming's over.

Thursday 20th January

Got a sweet text from Blog Boy checking we were still on for dinner when I get back from filming next week. His message was like a little shot of joy: I was standing outside for ten hours in the freezing rain today and knowing I have a date with him to look forward to really cheered me up.

Friday 21st January

I feel like a woman again. Finally I got some sex! I just couldn't wait any longer, despite all the texts from Blog Boy – my will power had evaporated.

And what a shag it was.

Last night Tony and I arranged to meet up after work in the hotel bar. We drank some wine, made some idle chit-chat about our day on set and then moved the conversation on to sex, Tony saying he hadn't had any for a while, me shyly agreeing, my pants already drenched.

It began to get late and with an early start this morning, we made our way to our rooms to go to bed, Tony stopping off at mine (supposedly) to 'compare' the room with his.

It didn't take long for things to happen: within minutes we were down to our underwear and were frantically grabbing at each other.

I finally got naked with a man for the first time in months.

I ripped off my pants and begged Tony to fuck me hard from behind as he bent me over the edge of the bed. He was just as charged up as me; he'd made me climax four times before even entering me. We both came together and I felt like months of frustration were relieved in one go.

Trying to work today with only one hour's sleep after all that action and then getting up at the crack of dawn wasn't really the best idea. I almost dropped a camera lens and got shouted at by my boss, which wasn't fun.

Plus I found out that Tony has a girlfriend. I can't believe he neglected to tell me that. If I had known, I would *never* have shagged him; I'm just not the kind of woman to be some bloke's 'bit on the side', nor do I want to be responsible for another woman being cheated on. I know how that feels. First Steven, now Tony: why do I seem to meet these arseholes? There must be some good men out there, who want to have some fun but aren't attached, surely?

Diary of a Sex Fiend

Monday 24th January

After a flurry of text messages over the last few days, I met up with Blog Boy again this evening at a lovely French restaurant in Soho. He looked even more irresistible this time. I could barely stop myself from looking at the curly chest hair that peeked over the open neck of his shirt. I wanted to run my fingers through it, but luckily I found some self-control from somewhere and kept my hands on the table where he could see them.

The thing is: I like him. I mean, I want to fuck him very much, but I also think he's a great guy. I can't help ticking off some of the boxes on my Potential Boyfriend Material check-list. Maybe it would be better to keep him on the backburner, for the future – when I've had some fun? Though given the opportunity of fucking him now, I don't think I could say no, especially since I spent most of the meal trying my best not to imagine him naked.

After we finished eating, he leaned over towards me and asked if he could kiss me. So I said yes; who am I to turn down a talented mouth artist who makes me squirm in my seat?

We snogged for ages, my hands somehow finding their way down his back, his around my waist. Finally the manager asked us to leave; it was past midnight and they wanted to shut the restaurant. Spoilsports.

We made our way to my bus stop, but got sidetracked on Oxford Street, his lips firmly pressed against mine, my hips firmly fixed against his.

'God, you're so sexy,' he said to me, as his hands slid underneath my top. 'You're a sexy, sexy girl, do you know that?'

I smiled at him shyly. 'Thanks,' I replied, and I gripped his arse tightly and pulled him closer to me, feeling his hardening cock against me as I did so. He grinned when he realised I could feel it too.

It wasn't long before his hands had wandered up under my skirt to rest on my bare arse (I do so love the combination of hold-up stockings and a thong). Thank God I was wearing a long coat – my skirt ended up hitched around my waist. We kissed and groped for ages, but once again I had to break it off – I had to be at the airport for my flight to New York in a few hours.

We walked on to my bus stop. 'See you when you get back in a week, yeah?' he asked.

'Definitely,' I replied and we kissed quickly once more, then I jumped on my bus and waved goodbye through the window as it pulled away, leaving him on the pavement.

And now I am sitting here drunk, horny and happy. I don't know what will happen with Blog Boy, but I can't wait to get to know him more.

It'll be difficult not to tear off his clothes and fuck him senseless when I get back from the States: I want to shag him rotten and I'm not sure if I'll be able to hold back next time I see him.

Tuesday 25th January

Finally on the way to New York, though my late-night dalliance with Blog Boy almost made me miss my plane. I'm sitting here scribbling about him instead of watching the in-flight, but I'm still excited about going to New York, even if it means I won't see him for a few days. It's been years since

I've seen my old friends in the Big Apple and I have a lot of catching up to do.

And maybe I'll even have a little fun while I'm over there, too.

Thursday 27th January

A girl never knows when horniness might strike. It could be at work, travelling on a bus, or during a business meeting. When it does kick in, you have three options:

1) **Ignore** the feeling and continue with what you were doing;
2) **Postpone** the feeling until you make it somewhere safe to play;
3) **Indulge** yourself there and then until your horniness is sated.

I found myself doing number three today in the lingerie section of Macy's department store. I tried very hard to keep quiet about it too.

It came out of the blue. I was trying on bras in the changing room, hoping to find something that would be simultaneously comfortable enough to wear to work *and* unbearably sexy to all who saw it. An ambitious wish, I know.

I was stripped down to my pants and doing the old *lift, hook and fasten* when I noticed that my nipples were erect, sticking out like bullets, even in the stifling temperature of the cubicle. I looked at my reflection and was struck by how hard they looked in the mirror. I pushed my hands into each cup of the bra and cradled my breasts, grazing my fingers against my nipples and feeling myself getting steadily more turned on.

It wasn't my reflection that was getting me steamed up; it was imagining what Blog Boy would see and do to me if *he* saw me so aroused, and that was making me wet.

I began to picture him standing behind me, his hands sliding up around my waist – like they'd been that night on Oxford Street – and then over my breasts, letting his fingers linger on the nipples, teasing them as he felt them growing firm under his touch. I went on cupping and squeezing my breasts in my hands as I fantasised about feeling his soft wet kisses on my bare skin. I pretended Blog Boy was behind me, pressing his body into mine, his rigid cock against me. When I pressed my fingers against my wet pants, I imagined it was his hand rubbing me, then pulling down my knickers and sliding himself into me.

I looked at myself squarely in the mirror. My pupils were dilated, my skin felt electric, my breath was heavy, and I was slippery with horniness. I began to rub harder, getting carried away, closing my eyes, faster now, then sliding a finger inside.

All of a sudden I heard 'Miss? Do you need any help in there? Did you try them all on yet?'

I suddenly remembered where I was – the lingerie section of a department store in New York City. The sales assistant wanted to give me some more bras to try on. She didn't know I was standing in front of the mirror with my hand between my legs. Not a good place to have a frig.

I was too far along and I had to finish what I'd started. With no other option, I threw my clothes on, grabbed my stuff and tried to find the ladies' room, but Macy's was huge; I ended up going up and down the escalators three times before I found a busy bathroom.

By the time I got there, I was throbbing, but I had to queue up with everyone else and wait my turn. I could have done with some sort of guest-list line for horny English girls, standing there with my pussy thrumming away like a fucking motor. At last I was in one of the stalls and set about preparing myself:

1) Remove iPod – check
2) Remove hat – check
3) Remove scarf – check
4) Remove coat – check
5) Remove jumpers (x2) – check
6) Pull down jeans – check
7) Pull down thermal leggings – check
8) Pull down pants (wet) – check
9) Slide hand in between legs – check
10) Notice the one-inch gap between the door and the wall – check

There's a *gap*? For some reason, in American public toilets, either side of the door there is a *gap* large enough to see into. I can't figure out if this is some government rule to prevent drug usage in public loos, or whether the people responsible for building these places were just bad at measuring up, but either way, it makes for a somewhat frustrating experience should you choose to masturbate in one of them.

So as well as having to *silently* frig myself into oblivion, I also had to position my body in such a way that I couldn't be *seen* through the gap either. A difficult task, yes, but I am pleased to report, not impossible. With the queue tapping their heels outside, I played to my heart's content, thinking about Blog Boy fucking me hard, and a short while later, all was well in my world.

And I managed to buy five bras after that too, so all in all, a good afternoon.

Sunday 30th January

Staying in Manhattan with Harry for the last few days has brought up a lot of old feelings. Five years older than me, I've known Harry since infancy. We are as close as siblings can be, without any of the rivalry you normally get between brothers and sisters. We love each other very dearly. When I was 17 our relationship changed and I fell in love with him. Although it's more than a decade since then, seeing him now, after two years in which we've barely spoken has reminded me how much I love and miss him.

Our closeness was always immediate, no matter how much time or geographical distance came between us. When I was little and he came round with his mum, we would be playing together within seconds, running off to have adventures in the park out of the grasp of our parents. Harry was the one who taught me how to roller-skate; he was this effortlessly cool older kid who I looked up to and learned from, and to him I was the sweet younger sister he never had.

So when I lived with him for some months during my seventeenth year, we shared a bed together – as we always had – and slept arm in arm, cuddling till we fell asleep. It all seemed normal, until one night altered everything.

I awoke to feel Harry's hand stroking my back. Nothing unusual; I turned towards him and sleepily draped my arm across his chest. We held each other for a minute. Even when his hand moved down towards my waist I thought nothing of it. It wasn't until his fingers slid under my right breast and began slowly caressing my nipple that I became aware that we were crossing a boundary. I felt Harry lift my breast gently, clasp it and then trace its outline with his index finger. I was conscious that my nipple was growing under his touch, and when he ran his thumb around it, it tingled enough to make me shiver.

We pressed closer to each other, I ran my hand across his chest. I remember hearing his breath quicken as the back of my hand touched his nipple. We looked at each other dreamily and began to kiss. It was so passionate, so gentle and so innocent. Our eyes were locked onto each other, we didn't need to say a word. It felt like the most natural thing in the world, even when Harry shifted and I could feel his cock against my thigh. Our bodies were in sync, our feelings expressed through this sexual closeness. We were two friends, hungrily searching and exploring each other, discovering the unknown parts of the other, adding to the love we already had.

So, we made love. It was amazingly intense, emotionally and physically. I truly loved him in every possible way and the time I spent with him all those years ago is something that to this day, I only recall fondly.

And now I find myself staying with him again, writing this diary entry at his very desk. A lot of years have passed since I was in love with Harry, some of them when we didn't get on so well, some when we didn't manage to see each other; our lives have become very separate.

But now I remember why I fell for him in the first place. Harry knows me almost better than I know myself. He'll say to me as we walk down the street together:

'Hey, Abby, you only tripped up once today, you're doing well so far!'

… And then grab me, because on cue, I've stumbled and am only saved from falling flat on my face by him catching me with perfect timing.

Harry knows what a messy person I am, how chaotic my house is and how much wine I manage to spill down my front. He'll point out:

'You missed a bit.'

And indicate my bust, where another new dark red stain has materialised, or he'll point out the accumulation of crumbs in my cleavage, and comment:

'Catch any more in there and you could start baking a cake.'

And I'll be laughing too hard to brush the crumbs out onto the floor. Harry knows how to make me crack up; I have actually wet myself because of something he said on more than one occasion.

Harry also knows I am a neurotic, overly analytical, slightly intense woman. He pulls me up on it all the time; tells me to calm down, stop thinking about things so hard and he tells me to:

'Just be yourself, everyone will love you.'

And I try. I do my best to rid myself of the pretentious bollocks that make up some of my defensive façade and just present myself as I am – take it or leave it. I pray that he's right: I hope there is someone out there that will see through the shit and wants me for who I am: clumsy git, cleavage-crumb-catcher and all.

Now that I'm staying with Harry yet again, I am loving his company. I'm feeling close to him once more, having missed his friendship for many years.

But now of course, we're no longer kids. He is a man. I am a woman. We have both grown up: he has a wife and a child, I have … well, a *different* life.

Looking at him now, I can still see how attractive he is. He has really grown into his mid-thirties self, no longer a cute boy but a handsome older man – beautiful laughter lines on his face, grey hairs on his head, podgier in his body. He is more relaxed now too, happier with himself and rid of the twenty-two-year-old's ego that I knew.

And even though I still find myself attracted to him, I am in no rush to ruin the friendship that we have managed to rebuild. There won't be any shagging between us. I am just enjoying being me with him, friendly, slightly flirtatious, and forever uncoordinated. I reckon that'll do me for the time being.

All that matters is that when I go home to London he's still my friend. Loving him and being loved in return, is more important than any sex I could have in the whole world. Almost makes me forget about Blog Boy. For a second.

Although I really do need a shag right now, it has to be said.

The Girl's Top Ten Guide

**How to respond to the sight of a single female
in a sex shop if you are a male customer:**

1 Do not blush or laugh at her. Certainly, do not approach her in the hardcore DVD section, point at particular titles and say, 'Done that, and that, *and that*. Think I'll get this one out again – got a real result from that.'

2 Do not stare at her wildly, amazed that women also wank and go shopping for sex material. We do.

3 Smile briefly and return to what you were doing. It's only polite and you are not there to chat her up after all.

4 Don't walk around with a hard-on. She won't be very impressed, even if you've got a large todger.

5 Try not to fill your shopping basket with a year's supply of porn. It'll just make you look desperate; a week's supply is more than enough.

6 Do not approach her with the largest dildo you can possibly find and then ask, 'What do you reckon, eh? Your type of thing?' Instead, have a look at the boys' toys and ask her what she thinks your girlfriend might like.

7 Stay away from the 'orifice' hardcore porn. Certainly spend no longer in the section than is necessary to 'tut' loudly and walk away shaking your head. No woman is impressed by a man who likes the sight of an anal canal held open and spread so widely that one can see right the way into it.

8 Do not laugh and joke with your mates in front of her about the porn actresses, saying, for example, 'Look at that one's fanny,' or 'What a slapper!' It's difficult enough for her to be in there, without being made to feel cheap, embarrassed or degraded.

9 Do not grab hold of her, demand to look through her basket and exclaim loudly in front of all your mates, 'She's got a huge dildo in there!'

10 Do peruse the 'couples' DVD section and the female sex toys, and ask the sales assistants for demonstrations to find out what gives women more stimulation.

This'll make you appear sensitive and generous, and will give women hope that not every man in a sex shop is a sad git who couldn't get laid if he tried. Plus, as well as giving you some idea of what women like, you might discover that you like it too …

2

February

Wednesday 2nd February

Back in London; exhausted, frustrated and horny, but happy. It was great to see my old friends in the Big Apple, especially Harry, whom I miss already.

Still, it's nice to be home; I'm really looking forward to seeing Blog Boy again, because it'll be our all-important third date – which should include a no-holds-barred shag if I've understood dating procedure correctly.

There's little doubt in my mind that if we continue where we left off last time, we'll end up jumping into bed together.

Whether we manage to eat a meal first is debatable.

Friday 4th February

My old school friend Kathy took me to a party tonight – one of her music industry do's. Odd how she mixes with all these superficial people on a daily basis, yet she hasn't changed since the day I met her when we were eleven. She's still an honest and caring person, regardless of the coked-up arseholes with whom she spends her daylight working hours.

After many cocktails I decided that there was zero talent

in the bar, so I told her about my mission to meet new men and have some fun. Kathy suggested that I try a singles' night, or speed dating – a perfect opportunity to find a guy who might be up for it, she reckoned.

Problem is, Kathy has a boyfriend and I don't know if I have the courage to go somewhere like that on my own. It's one thing chatting up a bloke but it's another thing altogether to have the guts to walk into a place and declare that you are free, single and gagging for a shag.

Even if it may be true.

Sunday 6th February

I am becoming aware that it doesn't take much to get me going at the moment. Seeing a handsome man sitting with his legs splayed apart on the tube set me off yesterday; observing the breast jiggle of a buxom woman as she ran for the bus gave me the shivers today; and I got very excited watching my neighbour get a blow job as he was preparing dinner this evening.

My neighbours have no blinds, bless them, so from the comfort of my own kitchen I have a perfect view of everything they get up to – not that I was sitting there in the dark with binoculars or anything. It's all on display to any who cares to watch, and that's how I found myself transfixed by the sight of my neighbour having his cock sucked by his boyfriend.

It started innocently enough. I happened to be idly look-ing out my window, enviously eyeing up their impressive jungle of houseplants. Obviously green-fingered, I was think-ing to myself, as I looked at the trailing boughs of ivy and ferns that hung all over the kitchen.

I spotted my neighbour Colin, framed by the greenery. His back was towards me and he was busy with a knife and chopping board and some vegetables. I debated whether I should ask him some gardening advice next time I saw him at the newsagent's, because I know I can kill a plant with a single glance (I am good with animals and children though, ironically).

Then his partner Simon walked in. He looked like he was tip-toeing up on Colin, creeping slowly into the room. I felt like I was privy to some dramatic moment – I couldn't wait to see how it turned out.

Simon edged slowly forwards. Colin continued chopping vegetables. And then, when Simon was only a foot away, he reached his arms around Colin and kissed his neck. I could see Colin laughing and he pushed his body up against Simon who held him tight.

It seemed like a nice warm embrace. I felt like I was intruding a little on their intimacy and was about to stop looking, when I suddenly saw Colin turn around and face Simon. In a split second, Simon was on his knees, had unzipped Colin's trousers and was sucking his cock furiously.

I was mesmerised. All I could do was watch with my heart pounding.

Simon sucking Colin deeply; Colin grinding his hips in towards Simon; Simon's hands on Colin's arse, pulling him in closer to his mouth.

God it was so erotic. Not only to see some form of real (non DVD-based) sex unfolding before my eyes, but also to observe a couple who were relaxed and free enough to drop everything and just have sex there and then. I wanted to cheer out loud for Simon when I saw that his way of saying hello to his lover was to surprise him with a blow job while he made the dinner – he was my kind of man.

This got me thinking about the monotony of having sex in the bedroom and how the familiarity and repetitiveness of our daily lives can manifest itself in the way we have sex with our partners. Who can honestly say they never get bored with the same old sleep, work, home, dinner, bed, shag routine? Sure, having sex outside the bedroom, or at other times of the day, helps to spice things up a little, but essentially what seems to be missing from the sexual experiences of those in long-term relationships is spontaneity. Even the sex between Steven and I – as great as it was – became somewhat routine.

So this spur of the moment blow job has made me realise: it's not so much *when* you have sex that matters, as *what you are doing when you do it*. By treating his partner to some oral sex while he was cooking, Simon ensured that not only the sex, but also the chore at hand – dicing carrots – was made more interesting and exciting. The next time Colin chops vegetables, I bet he gets a hard-on.

Now I'm wondering how I'd incorporate this philosophy into my own sex life. I'm thinking:

★ A guy ironing some shirts. I walk up behind him, kiss his neck, caress his nipples, slide a hand down the front of his jeans and grip his cock.
★ Me washing up. A man comes up behind me, squeezes my breasts, lifts my dress, bends me over the sink and slides his dick into me.
★ A bloke dusting the ceiling. When he reaches up, I pull down his zipper and draw his penis into my mouth.

All these scenarios have this in common: they incorporate sex spontaneously and with regularity into a domestic routine. Both the domestic and the sexual regime get sparked up as a result.

The only drawback I can see is that chores might take slightly longer than normal to complete, given the need for a brief shagging interval. However, in the short term there're orgasms and in the long term a healthy sex life, so the temporary shortfall in housework seems worth it.

If there's the incentive of getting wet soapy tits when you're bent over the sink and taking a good, hard cock from behind, then I may just be persuaded to do some washing-up after all.

I *really* need to hear from Blog Boy soon.

Thursday 10th February

Finally got a text from Blog Boy saying hello. It's been over a week since I got back from New York and we still haven't arranged when to meet up for our third date.

I know he's busy at the moment, but surely with the heat we generated, he wants to meet up too?

I know I shouldn't read anything into this apart from the fact that he's tied up with his career, but it would be nice if he worked a little harder to make sure we meet up again.

I'm really craving a shag right now and if he doesn't fix something up soon, I may just have to find someone else.

Saturday 12th February

I can't stop thinking about men's cocks. I've been busily checking out men's crotches on the street, hoping to God I haven't been caught looking, and have decided that one of the sexiest things in the world is to be able to see the shape of an erect cock pressed up against the material of a guy's trousers. It's glorious.

If he wasn't wearing any underwear, that would be even better. Is there anything sexier than being able to trace the outline of a swollen cock through a pair of jeans? I think not.

Don't get me wrong; I am a huge fan of the naked erect member, as much as, if not more than, the next girl. I wish I could worship some gorgeous specimens of manhood right now. It's just that I've come to appreciate the thought of seeing a cock straining up against a man's fly buttons. I loved it that night when Blog Boy's jeans ended up being a mini-prison for him, his penis aching to get out from behind the 'bars' of his trousers.

Seeing that bulge – that growing form – battling for space in the trouser department was like a drug to me; it's no wonder that I was so wet when I felt Blog Boy pressing against me in the street.

I suppose it was because I couldn't have immediate access to his cock; that little obstacle made me want him all the more. To know, to see, to feel, that he was hard, but not be able to imme-diately touch him – flesh to flesh – made me crazy. Like one of Pavlov's dogs I started to salivate, a miniature waterfall began in my pussy, and I was filled with an uncontrollable desire to eat, to slide his cock into my mouth and gobble it all up hungrily. Yum.

So you see, with this in mind, when I think about some of the ways that a bloke might express himself, I would be quite happy for him not to bother with boring flowers, chocolates or lingerie if he wants to get in my pants/apologise/impress me. All he needs is a sharp intellect, the ability to make me laugh, and have a dirty enough mind to know that his half-hidden rigid cock will have me begging to be fucked by him pronto.

And have a button-fly on his jeans: I wouldn't want to cause any damage when I rip them off him.

Monday 14th February

Tom texted me today:

'I may be in your neck of the woods soon. Feel like some fun?'

It's been a year since I've seen Tom; our last meeting consisted of some rampant drunken shagging. We both met other people after that and he went back up to Birmingham, so I removed him from my 'possibility list'.

Maybe he's single now?

I texted to find out.

'Are you being a naughty boy?'

He responded straight away:

'No, we broke up; it's all fine. But I'm horny as hell – want to hook up when I'm in London in a few weeks?'

'Yes,' I replied, somewhat eagerly, 'Buzz me when you're about.'

Fantastic: if Blog Boy doesn't come through, I may have another shag lined up instead. Hurrah. I guess it is a Happy Valentine's Day after all.

Wednesday 16th February

I have an addiction. I tell myself I won't let it get the better of me, but it is officially out of my control. No, not the sex one.

The other one. You see, I now have almost one hundred items of underwear in my drawer.

I know it is not normal to make regular purchases of slinky pants, lacy basques or satin suspender belts, but I can't stop myself. Every time I am in a clothing store I find myself in the lingerie department, fondling some soft, sensual material, thinking how cute it would look with my arse in it, or clinging to my breasts, and before I know it, my credit card is being swiped and said item is whisked into a bag and taken back home. Needless to say, I bought far too many knickers when I was in New York.

And now I have just found a new sexy pair of knickers in my drawer that I don't even recall buying: this habit is really getting too much.

There are pants of every style you could imagine in there: tiny g-string thongs, hipster hot-pants, fitted briefs, tie-string shorts, satin, silk, Lycra, cotton, lace, mesh, and of course every conceivable colour. I haven't even started on the basques, the teddies or the suspender belts.

I'm not sure when this addiction started. For years I wasn't into wearing anything *saucy*, because I thought I would just be perpetuating the same sexist, objectified view of femaleness that was shoved down my throat by the cover of every magazine.

Back then I thought that wearing lingerie represented the male fantasy of female sexual availability, so how could a feminist like me wear something that seemed to exist just to turn a man on? Plus, the thought of my partner getting off on me wearing frilly underwear made me extremely uncomfortable, so all my early relationships were spent wearing *comfortable* knickers and *sensible* bras. Bridget Jones had nothing on my big pants.

At some point in the last couple of years, I began to find lingerie appealing. I started to enjoy looking at it and touching it, and when I held it against my skin, it made me feel seductive. The biggest shock came when I finally slipped a lacy g-string up my thighs and the sight of the curve of my arse against the material turned me on, making me want to touch myself.

So I did. My hands followed the line of the thong as it reached down between my legs; the material felt delicate against my skin, and, my fingers didn't take long to slide underneath the lacy fabric and rub me to oblivion. You could say it was a watershed moment. From then on I began to revise my anti-lingerie stance.

Surely there was nothing wrong with wearing something that made me feel so sexy? And I found out that it also turned me on to know that I could turn on a partner too: I liked the idea that a man could enjoy a thing that gave me so much pleasure – even if it was the thought of me in a boned basque and stockings. I didn't feel degraded by this, I felt empowered.

Fast forward to now, and I cannot bloody stop myself from purchasing lingerie. Because I'm single most of my pants don't even see the light of day, let alone get the chance of being fondled by another person, so I have no idea why I keep on buying more.

Recent purchases include:

★ Baby-blue satin low-rider hipsters with black piping
★ Black lacy French knickers with a 'v' plunging in the front
★ Bright pink satin thong
★ Lilac shorts with black lace trim
★ And my favourites: black satin briefs with a slit cut out in the rear, held together (just) with three pink bows

However, I'm not going to try any of these on in front of my mirror: that'd be a waste of perfectly clean pants, because my hand would wander down *just* to test out how silky the material really was and then …

No, I think I shall save these for a *special* day, for a *special* somebody to appreciate. And to wrestle them off me.

I hope that happens soon though; I haven't got many *normal* pants to wear until then.

Friday 18th February

I don't know if it is because:

a)   my wank last night didn't fulfil me totally
b)   I have only had three hours' sleep
c)   I have had no time to play with myself today due to work

– but I knew it was going to be tough for me tonight when I was soaking wet before I even got on the tube.

I was meeting my mate Tim for drinks. We met at college and have known each other for more than a decade now, but there's no sex on the agenda any more – we're just friends, which is great.

It was different when we first met: we shagged with a passion, but both decided we'd be better off as mates. Getting the sex stuff out of the way helped us become much closer, and we can now talk very honestly about sex, which is wonderful: it has helped us both to get the other gender's perspective on it all.

So, a bottle of wine drunk and we're both merry, talking about shagging. Tim's been having a dry patch too, but that has recently changed, due to his hot new fuck-buddy (lucky bastard).

He told me about their third meeting:

'So I knock on her door and she opens it.'

Me: 'What's she wearing?'

Him: 'Does it matter?' *(He sees my disappointed look.)* 'Oh, OK, a tight top and a short skirt. So, anyway, I walk in, shut the door behind me, and say to her, "bend over".'

Me: 'And?'

Him: 'And she bends over. I walk up to her and I can see she has no underwear on.'

Me: 'Oh fuck! What did you do? Stick it in her?'

Him *(grinning)*: 'No. That's what she was expecting, and I didn't want her to take me for granted. So I lifted her skirt up and started licking her instead.'

Me *(clapping my hands in glee)*: 'Ha! You bad boy! And?'

Him: 'Oh, you know, I stuck my tongue inside her and she went crazy, started begging me to stick my cock in ...'

Me: 'And did you? Please tell me you did, you cruel bastard ...'

Him: 'Yeah. I walked her over to the couch, bent her over again, pulled up her skirt and slid it in.'

Me: 'I bet she came straight away ...'

Him *(proudly)*: 'Of course, but she came even harder when I slapped her arse cheeks and fingered her hole.'

Me: 'Mmm ...'

So we're sitting there, drunk, and I am thinking:

★ Tim is my good mate
★ We are friends
★ Sex would fuck things up

41

★ We have put our sexual history together behind us

★ I am not that attracted to him

But, I was also SO fucking worked up. The whole time he was describing his shag I was getting jealous – wishing that it was Blog Boy in front of me so I could just jump him, and I was getting wetter and wetter.

I regretted not having had time to play with myself before I went out to meet Tim; leaving the house with a throbbing pussy is a dangerous thing for me to do right now.

My rational brain began to shut down. I started thinking about getting out of my seat and walking over to Tim to say:

'You don't mind if I sit on your lap for a minute, do you? It's OK if I just rest my legs here, isn't it, how about I wrap them around your hips?

'You want to know why that is? I am just a little hot, that's all. Yes, that's good. What's that? I have no underwear on? Oh dear, I must have forgotten to put some on, silly me.

'Comfortable now, isn't it? You can feel something damp? That'd be me, I do apologise; how about I rub myself against you and let you absorb some of my wetness?

'No need to apologise, I like that pressing into me, let me just hoist myself up a little – that's better. Maybe you should place your hands around my thighs for stability. Actually, I meant the inside of my thighs. What? They are wet? Well, maybe you should rub your fingers all around there, wouldn't want an accident there, would we?

'Now, how about we unzip that fly, get your cock out and slide it deeply into me, hmm? We could talk about that movie we saw last week; no need to discuss the juices flowing out of me as you fuck me with your hard cock, now, is there?'

And so on …

I sat there, pussy pulsing away, soaking wet, stupidly tempted to throw away our friendship for one quick randy moment.

But destiny intervened: Tim's fuck-buddy called and wanted to meet up immediately, so we said our goodbyes and went our separate ways.

And now I sit here, with another great friend of mine: my favourite vibrator. May our friendship continue indefinitely.

Sunday 20th February

Still no response from Blog Boy to a text I sent him yesterday. I know I'm getting neurotic, but not replying for more than 24 hours seems suspicious to me. Maybe he has gone off me?

Why am I bothered that he might have?

Monday 21st February

Blog Boy finally replied to my text. Seems he's still busy with work. Pretty feeble response, I guess, but I know what it's like. When I have work, everything else falls by the wayside.

Anyway, he suggested meeting for a meal next week, so I guess the interest is still there, and no, I still wouldn't turn down a shag with him.

Fingers crossed something happens; if all goes to plan, my new sexy knickers will get an airing at last.

Diary of a Sex Fiend

Saturday 26th February

I have come to the conclusion that I must be a size queen. I admit it: I like large men. In fact, more than that, I *adore* large men, and when faced with someone big like Blog Boy, it's no wonder that I swoon (and drip) in his presence.

Penis-size, however, I really couldn't give two shits about; as long as the owner of said cock knows how to use it well, then the fact that it's large or small makes no difference to me whatsoever.

No, my size issue is different altogether. It regards the main three physical attributes of a man – besides the face, eyes and arse of course – that grab my attention and make me go weak at the knees:

1) if he is tall
2) if he has large hands
3) if he has big feet

Now, my liking of these things is not some kind of fetish, but it is fair to say that they all form part of the somewhat idiosyncratic requirements that I have of a man.

Regarding height:

I am not being discriminatory against short men for sexual reasons. I'm not saying that short men are incapable of satisfying me – I have dated men shorter than myself in the past and been perfectly well served. It's just that given my outgoing and somewhat dominant personality, it takes a lot of man to make me feel all girly and shy. Being with someone whose sheer physical presence – his height – overpowers my own size,

44

leaves me feeling like a smitten kitten, curled up safe in the arms of her protector, or being made to meow for her dinner. Either way, purring loudly.

So I need my man to be taller than me: the taller the better, six foot minimum. I want to feel that I am small and girly. I want to get a tired neck from leaning up to kiss him. And I want the reason I am staggering about in five-inch heels is so that I can feel his cock between my legs when we embrace.

Regarding hand size:

I don't just think, I *know* that it's a total myth that there is a correlation between hand and cock size – Tony had quite small hands and a large cock, whilst Steven had huge hands and a tiny cock – so my earlier, uninformed assumptions about the two being connected have been proved wrong.

But regardless of cock size, for me, a man must have large hands. Small ones not only do not turn me on: they actively turn me off.

Now this is partly due to the outsize 'man-hands' (as Kathy and Fiona put it) that I myself have – my un-dainty, non-frag-ile-looking, big mitts dwarf all the female hands that I encounter and, quite often, male ones too. Naturally I have an issue with this – an insecurity if you will. After all, I couldn't bring myself to shag a man whose breasts were larger than my own 36 double Ds, so how could I feel all feminine and sexy when his *petites mains* looked slight and delicate next to mine?

There's another reason for my hand-fascism. When I saw Blog Boy and his large hands, I could only think of one thing: his lovely long fingers inside me, filling me up. It's just not the same with short stubby fingers.

Sod having a big cock, I want big fingers to fuck me. I

want to feel that he owns me with his hands, that when his fingers are inside me, it feels like my pussy belongs to him. And when he motions with his forefinger to 'come hither' that it means exactly that: 'Get your arse over here, Abby – you see these big fingers? They're going to stroke you until you drench my hand with your juices.' Whoever thought that just beckoning me towards them would make me wet? But it does.

Regarding foot size:

I have one rule here. It has nothing to do with wanting his toes inside me, having a hard kick on my butt, or licking his feet – though possibly the first one might be interesting to try, now that I think about it. Nor does it have anything to do with cock size, any other kind of penetration, or anything else sex-related.

It comes down to this: I have size eight and a half feet, so I think I should never date a man with feet smaller than my own. Shallow, I know. But since I am a vain cow, then in order to make my feet look dainty and feminine – which, let's face it, is every woman's objective when she is wearing a pair of stilettos – then my partner has to have damn huge feet.

No one, I repeat no one, is going to make me feel like a fucking, massive duckfooted-boat-impersonating-heffalump.

Though I suppose that if he were six foot four with massive hands, I might make an exception.

But he'd have to be really good in the sack.

And not try on my shoes when I was out at work.

The Girl's Guide to Cock Size

Small

Pros	Cons
You can get fucked as hard as you like	It doesn't always fill you up
It always rubs the g-spot	It doesn't push against your cervix
The length of it can lie against your labia with the tip tickling your clit	Sometimes you can't feel it inside you
You can rub it through jeans without it being noticeable	It doesn't always show through jeans when hard
You can get it all in your mouth without choking	Sometimes it's nice to deep-throat
Easier to give a hand job – if it only fits into one fist	Using only fingers to stroke it can be frustrating
Holding it when standing can make you feel powerful	Penetrative sex whilst standing up is often difficult
It feels wonderful inside your arse	It can be difficult finding a good angle of entry

Large

Pros	Cons
It fills you up and you feel like you are getting 'fucked'	Being filled up can hurt and prevent you getting fucked hard
It pushes against your cervix and stimulates your womb	A constant pushing against your cervix can be painful and annoying
It tugs on your labia during penetration and thus indirectly stimulates your clit	It can rub your labia too intensely, making you sore
It looks beautiful when hard underneath jeans	Hiding an erection under clothing is difficult
It gives you deep orgasms	It misses your g-spot
You can feel like a girl when you hold it, or put it in your mouth	It can be more laborious to give a hand job and you can't get it all in your mouth
It can reach any position, any angle, any depth	Not all positions can be comfortable
It makes you feel intimidated and excited	Forget about anal: no chance that is gonna fit in there, mate

3

March

Wednesday 2nd March

Finally met up with Blog Boy again this evening – the notorious third date. It wasn't the ideal time to meet because I had done an exhausting 14-hour day and was very tired, but he was booked solid for the next few months and I knew I'd have too much work on my plate then as well, so I didn't want to let this chance slip by and lose all that momentum.

Plus I was gagging for a shag.

So even though I was dressed in work clothes, my hair was a mess, I had no make-up on and I looked as knackered as I felt, I drove straight from work to meet him for a late dinner. Fuck it, I thought, he's going to have to see me looking rough at some point – better for him to see the real me and not just think of me as the sexy, sultry girl who let him grab her arse in the middle of Oxford Street.

It was great to see him again; we caught up on each other's lives, ate some lovely food in a tapas bar and laughed a lot. It felt like hardly any time had passed since we last met; there was no embarrassment or awkward silences between us. The rapport was instant.

So when I drove him home a couple of hours later and leaned over the steering wheel to kiss him, I was shocked that he then pulled away and said, 'I'd prefer it if we were just friends from now on, if that's OK with you.'

I was speechless; I really didn't see that coming. All I could do was mumble that it was 'fine with me; friends is great', before driving off in a state of shock.

I was so stunned by what he had said that I got hopelessly lost driving home. The journey took me twice as long as it should have because I was racking my brain to try to understand why he would suddenly be so disinterested in me, after seeming so keen.

And now I am sat here, unable to sleep for my confusion. I thought he liked me – how could I get it so wrong? I know it's silly, but I can't help but feel gutted that he's fobbed me off with the whole 'friends' thing; I thought at the very least he wanted to sleep with me.

Friday 4th March

The Blog Boy episode seems to have ended in frustration and Tom's been sending me loads of flirty text messages that lead nowhere, so I decided to call him and see if he was in town. It's about time we had another shag.

'Hey, Abby,' Tom said as he answered the phone, 'Nice to hear from you! How are things?'

'Not bad,' I replied. 'Been a while, eh?'

He laughed. 'Yeah, maybe too long. Work going well?'

'Fine,' I said, 'but I haven't called you to talk about work.'

There was a pause. 'Why did you call me then?' Tom asked.

'I think you know,' I said, slowly.

'No, I don't. Tell me.'

'Well,' I said, trying to find the words, 'I think there are better things to do with my mouth than talk all night.'

Tom laughed again, 'And what might that be, Abby?'

I took a deep breath and swallowed my shyness. 'Sliding your cock between my lips and sucking it deeply?'

I heard him breathe heavily. 'Well, in that case, maybe you need to jump straight in a cab and come over; I'm staying in Westbourne Park.' His voice sounded gruff.

'Yes, I think that's a good idea,' I replied, and was relieved that I had already showered, shaved my legs and put on a new pink lacy thong just minutes before calling him. I do like to be prepared.

Later, when I arrived at Tom's, we did end up having a conversation – of sorts:

'I forgot how hard you come, Abby,' he gasped, as my convulsions subsided for a moment. 'When you come, you COME, eh?'

'Mmm,' I replied, as I shifted back up to face him, my breasts in front of his mouth.

He began kissing my nipples again, and tugged them gently. I slid my legs around him and tucked my ankles behind his arse. We moved together for a while.

'God, you're close again, I can *feel* you,' he breathed in my ear, as I gripped his back and held on for dear life.

'Fuck … that feels *good*.' My toes curled and my insides began to grip him like a vice.

He pulled me closer, holding my shaking hips as he slid me up and down his cock. We paused for a second and I caught my breath once more.

'Right. Let's try something else.' He picked me up and flipped me over so that just my back lay on the couch. He knelt on the floor and pushing my knees back towards my chest, rested my ankles on his shoulders. Then he slid himself into me sharply and I trembled.

'Mmm, you're off again!' he said, as he grabbed my tits and began thrusting. I quivered, dug my hands into his arse cheeks and gripped his neck with my toes, my body tensing up.

'Jesus. Fuck me. Harder ...' I trailed off, almost unaware of his groaning, grimacing and steady pumping as I spasmed away uncontrollably.

'Fucking hell, what's with you tonight? You're on fire!' Tom said as he picked me up once again and sat himself back down on the couch, ensuring he was still inside me as I slid my legs around him.

'It just feels ... so good ... ooh ...' I pushed myself onto him deeply, and rode him again.

'Yeah, go on, yeah,' he moaned, as I clawed my nails into his back. 'Ouch!'

'Sorry,' I murmured, and slid my hands around his neck, holding him tightly as my convulsions started up again.

He grasped my arse and pulled me into him as the waves of pleasure filled me once more. 'That was sudden. Where did that one come from, eh?'

(To him): 'I think it was your cock rubbing against my g-spot. It felt so fucking good.'

(To myself): I can't quite believe it, but I think that the excitement of fucking to the band Kasabian's song 'Reason Is Treason' made me come. How weird is that?

We waited a moment for my shivering to subside. Then he pushed me off him and stood up, cock still rigid. 'Right. There's something I've been waiting to try.'

He motioned me to walk round to the end of the couch.

I slowly managed to manoeuvre my still-shaking body there and stood next to the waist-high arm.

'Bend over,' he said, and leaned me over the arm so that my upper body was draped downwards into the seat of the couch. I grabbed hold of the sofa cushion as he slipped himself into me.

'Mmmfghrbmmm ...' I mumbled, as he began to thrust, my mouth pressed up against the cushion.

'Uuugh,' he groaned, holding my hips and pumping me hard from behind. My legs began to shake once more. They felt like jelly. I clung onto the cushion for dear life.

'Uh, fuck, yeah!' he panted, 'Jesus, I can feel you coming again! Fuck!'

I heard myself saying (through the cushion): 'Harder. Harder. Fuck me. Oh God, please. Harder!' and I ground my teeth, went blind, lost control of my legs and shuddered violently.

Our convulsions were simultaneous. He pulled out, removed the condom and sat down on the sofa, but I couldn't move. All feeling in my legs was gone. The only sensation I had was of my body quivering like a jellyfish. I was still clinging to the sofa cushion to stop myself collapsing; I just couldn't stop trembling.

'Been a while, has it?' he asked, laughing and out of breath.

I grinned at him through my post-coital haze; if only he knew.

Monday 7th March

I am ill. My throat hurts, my lungs ache and I feel groggy.

Ever since I got back from shagging Tom, I've been sat

under the duvet feeling sorry for myself. Not even a little fiddle here and there makes me feel better – which says a lot.

Earlier I had to venture out to my local supermarket to do a quick shop and get some emergency essentials. Even with a crappy cough and bunged-up head, I had to brave it and stock up on food and groceries.

Oddly, two guys proceeded to have the following conversation about me down one of the supermarket aisles:

Male #1 after having walked past me three times to check me out (to Male #2): 'Well, *would* you?'

Male #2 (loud enough for me to hear; looking at my arse): 'I *would*.' He smiled at me and then looked at the curve of my breasts against my t-shirt. 'With *pleasure*.'

Male #1 nodded in affirmation. He joined Male #2 in the dairy section, and they grinned at me.

At that precise moment, my flu decided it would be the absolute perfect time to exit my body in a retching, loud, throttling hacking that can only be compared to the sound of an antelope having its throat bitten into by a leopard and choking out its final breath.

Not sexy; especially not with added sputum. While I was busy hacking a good ole phlegm-filled cough (with a massive sneeze too, for added sensuality) the boys scarpered, and I can't blame them really. I am not at my sexiest with a runny nose, it has to be said.

Although, thinking about it, when I was round at Tom's, I was literally dripping onto him. And not only from down below. No, clearly I was just developing the beginnings of the flu and my nose was running like a tap when we were shagging – no amount of tissues could dry it up.

But Tom didn't seem to mind: he just pulled me down

onto his cock, gripped me harder and told me, 'A good shag'll bring it out of you.'

Amen to that.

Tuesday 8th March

I got an email from Blog Boy today.

In it, he tried to explain that though he liked me and was attracted to me, he just wasn't ready to be in a relationship right now, because he wanted to travel in the summer and his job-hopping didn't leave space for someone else in his life.

He apologised if he misled me in any way by showing so much interest, but wanted to let me know that he was trying to do the 'right thing' by not acting on his attraction to me and asking to be friends instead.

But when I then emailed back and suggested we have a fling instead – there's always hoping – he wrote back immediately and said he didn't want us to be fuck-buddies, because he wasn't good at casual sex. Plus he was worried that if we did get involved, that he might end up hurting me, so he wanted to put a stop to things before they developed any further.

He reassured me that he meant what he said about staying friends; that we should meet up soon for dinner, that he really enjoyed my company.

I am really pleased he came clean; at least I know I wasn't imagining the whole thing, and the fact that he respected me enough to NOT fuck me, because he wants to ensure we stay friends, says a lot about him. It's nice to know that he thinks of me as more than just a potential fuck-buddy.

Though that doesn't stop me wanting to shag him rotten.

Diary of a Sex Fiend

Saturday 12th March

Given the Blog Boy situation, I finally decided to take up Kathy's suggestion of going to a singles' evening at a club last night. And as luck would have it, I actually managed to meet someone there.

Not that I had planned to; I had dragged Kathy, who's perfectly happy with her boyfriend, along to the Gardening Club in Covent Garden as moral support. I promised her there would be free cocktails if she'd come and keep me company while I checked out the talent and got more confident about my chat-up technique.

I certainly didn't expect to be going to some cheap hotel afterwards and trying out *hand-job* techniques on a complete stranger, but after a few drinks, when I spotted him standing by the bar, I just knew I had to talk to him. Tall, with baby-blue eyes, unkempt fair hair and large hands, he was just my type.

So I plucked up all my courage and made my way over to him, catching his eye in the mirror and smiling shyly at him. To my relief, he smiled back and we began chatting quite easily.

Ben was from Manchester and down in London on business; he mentioned that he had ended up in the bar because he was trying to have a drink somewhere near his hotel. I noted this information keenly: very handy, I thought, nice and local.

We talked and drank for a couple of hours, our conversation getting more flirtatious as time went on. At some point Ben's hand subtly landed on my knee and I knew that things were looking good.

When I placed my hand on his knee in response, he looked down at it and then grinned at me, saying,

'Maybe we should go to my hotel and have a quieter drink there?'

I didn't need much persuading: it was getting harder to concentrate on the conversation as I got more and more aroused.

So I went over to Kathy who was busy schmoozing with the DJ and told her it looked like I could have got lucky. She laughed, wished me luck and demanded that I call her first thing tomorrow with details. I promised her I'd fill her in and she gave me a friendly slap on the arse as I rejoined Ben and we made our way to his hotel.

We didn't waste much time when the door was shut behind us; our clothes were off in seconds and our hands all over each other. Almost before I knew it, his fingers were inside me and I was climaxing over and over again. He was very skilled in that department, that's for sure.

It was then that I felt a little inadequate. Jerking a guy off has got to be the part of sex I am least sure about; to be able to pleasure a man just by stroking his cock is a big achievement in my eyes. I almost felt unqualified to touch him after his skilful display.

The reason I'm not so confident about it is because years ago, when I was 16, I was enthusiastically tugging away at Danny's member when he remarked,

'You're not very good with your hands, are you?'

Needless to say, it made me self-conscious and nervous about touching a man's penis for *quite* a while.

So up until last night I was still nervous about giving a guy a good hand job. I was terrified that he might go soft as I stroked him – a clear indication of poor technique, I presumed. I couldn't bear the thought that my incompetence would turn him off that much.

But Ben was a complete stranger and I knew that if it all

went horribly wrong, I wouldn't have to worry about seeing him again, so I thought I should maybe give it a try.

And, well, I've been doing some research on-line, and there's a lot of information out there on giving good hand jobs. I absorbed everything I could find that had anything to do with putting your hands on male genitals. If it was about tickling perineums, I wanted it. Ball-squeezing, I wanted it. Even prostate stimulation. I wanted to know it all.

Until now all I've needed is someone to *practise* on.

And there was Ben, lying on the hotel bed with a raging hard-on. Perfect.

I got myself ready.

That is, I pulled out the sachet of lube that I have been carrying around in my purse and squirted a generous amount onto my hands.

I have read that lube is essential for a good hand job: by adding some slick, slippery wetness, it would make my hands feel like a pussy gripping his cock, and that was precisely the effect I was aiming for.

I sat astride his legs, his erect penis just in front of me between my thighs and I reached down with my right hand to take a hold of it. I started off really slowly, making sure my well-lubed fingers caressed every bump and ridge as they moved up and down his cock.

He loved it. Really. I was amazed at the response. His cock was rock hard in my hands, his balls tightly tucked up underneath, and he was grinding his hips up towards me and groaning loudly.

So that move worked, hooray! But why stop there? He may have wanted to come but I wanted to try out all my new tricks on him, so try them out I did.

I intertwined my fingers, as if I was praying (to the God of Cock – the only deity I believe in) and I slid his cock between my palms. He most certainly enjoyed that. I even got to see the whites of his eyes as he thrashed about on the bed.

I wouldn't let him come yet, and I started to enjoy teasing him: he was on the brink many times and I would keep slowing down to allow him to catch his breath before starting up again, faster.

Eventually I decided to go all out: I stroked Ben up and down, with one hand, and with the other I held his balls first, then tugged them gently, moved on to stroking his perineum, and then, finally, sliding my slippery index finger into his arsehole, stroked his prostate lightly as he moved his body back and forth against my hand.

I've never seen a guy come so intensely – the force, the spurting, the entire body clenching up – and he gritted his teeth as he let out this animal noise and climaxed. It was wonderful. I had no idea that he would enjoy it so much; my homework had paid off!

Ben then made me come again and I relaxed, knowing that I had mastered the hand job at last.

I can't wait to try out my new manoeuvres on another guy now.

Sunday 13th March

The hand-job triumph set me thinking about a one-night stand I had a few years ago, which ended up in another kind of hand job altogether – one that was considerably less satisfying.

I met Rick through film work; we had been on the same

project for a couple of weeks and got on well together … He was a gentle, intelligent soul, with a mind as dirty as my own. Naturally I was smitten; I thought he was definitely Potential Boyfriend Material.

At the wrap party, plied by much alcohol, things finally stepped up a gear. He called me over to him on the dance floor, placed a hand on my shoulder and asked me,

'What do you think of masturbation?' and then grinned at me widely, not a bit coy.

I pondered on this for a moment before I replied as truthfully as I could.

'Well, I think it's great; I rather enjoy it in fact.'

He laughed. 'No, I meant, what do you think of guys masturbating? You know, watching them do it?'

Again I thought it best to be truthful. I leant into him and said softly in his ear, 'I think it's lovely, it's like seeing the most intimate thing a guy could do.'

His expression changed and he stared at me fixedly. 'Does it turn you on, then?' he asked.

'Very much so,' I practically whispered, as he leant in towards me and planted a soft kiss on my lips.

Thirty minutes later we were sitting in the starkly lit living room of his shared house, refuelling our drunken bodies with more beer. We sat at opposite ends of the couch, not so confident now we were out of the dingy nightclub.

After a while he broke the silence: 'Do you mind if I play with myself?'

I was a little stunned and mumbled something incoherent, feeling myself blush at his forwardness.

'Would you mind if I masturbated?' he repeated, 'Seeing you sitting there looking so gorgeous is really turning me on.'

Well, who was I to refuse such a polite request? I agreed, and he immediately pulled out his cock and began to stroke it.

With a mixture of apprehension, curiosity and horniness, I watched him play with himself. It was absolutely gripping – so to speak – I was transfixed by the sight of this man gazing at me, and pleasuring himself.

I felt my nervousness begin to disappear as I got increasingly aroused. I moved to his side of the couch, swung my hips over him, pushed my breasts into his face and kissed him deeply. We moved together for a while, tugging at each other's clothes, then stumbled half dressed into his bedroom.

He peeled off all his clothes and laid me on my back, telling me to play with myself. Then he knelt between my legs, his cock in his own fist, watching me. As he fondled himself, I began to lose my inhibitions and started to stroke myself too. It was very intense and intimate: our hands moving in synchronisation as we pleasured ourselves.

When he came the first time, all over my belly, it felt like we were connected and his enjoyment was part of something between us. We relaxed and snogged a bit, and I thought about how much I liked him. Then he started to masturbate again.

When he came the second time, all over my thighs, I felt a little disappointed. I had wanted to have penetrative sex, but he kept saying 'Isn't safe sex the best!' as he yanked away, grabbing my breasts with his spare hand, so I didn't say anything.

When he came the third time, all over my tits, I felt used. I was no longer a girl he wanted to be intimate with, or get to know, I was just there to help him get off. Wank fodder, basically. He didn't even look at me as he orgasmed, and he didn't seem bothered about whether I was having fun or not.

Maybe it was all the alcohol, but I couldn't orgasm. I had

too many thoughts running through my head. I liked him, but now suspected that I was just an easy fuck as far as he was concerned. I decided to test the water, and in my non-assertive way, I mildly hinted at our meeting up again, and offered my phone number.

He fobbed me off with a vague 'of course we'll hook up' and 'you know how to get hold of me', before drifting off to sleep and snoring loudly. He may have liked me before, but now he had got me into bed, he didn't want me any more.

As I lay there, wide awake with my thoughts, I was filled with self-hatred and regret. I felt like I had ruined a perfectly good opportunity for something to develop by allowing desire to rule my head and jumping into bed with him far too quickly.

As he lay next to me, I felt terribly alone. All I wanted was to get out of there, to stop the conflict in my head and the pounding in my heart.

I waited for the dawn to arrive, and when it did, I quietly put on my clothes, grabbed my bag and crept to the door. As I opened it I heard 'Not even going to leave me a note, then?' and I turned to see him sitting up in bed looking at me.

I walked back over to him and made some excuse about having to leave early to prepare for a meeting. He ran his hand around my back and down to my arse, giving it a gentle squeeze.

'Come back to bed,' he coaxed, 'I'm already hard thinking about you.'

So he had 'morning wood' and was looking for a way to get off. I fancied him, and I wanted to fuck him, but I wanted more than to be just his masturbatory fantasy. If that was all he wanted from me, I wasn't going to stay there and let him wank over me again.

So I said my goodbyes and left.

We barely spoke again after that; I saw him on a few different jobs and we avoided each other.

Although this experience wasn't great, it did help me learn a lot about having casual sex: a one-night stand is all fine, good and a lot of fun, just so long as that is *all* you want from that person. Don't embark on casual sex with someone that you want a relationship with.

Even if the thought of them naked makes you wet.

Thursday 17th March

I have discovered that my arms are too short.

★ Not too short to lift a cocktail glass to my lips and sip my drink elegantly
★ Not too short to wave flirtatiously at the handsome man who smiled at me today
★ Not too short to wipe the sweat from my brow as I try to beat my five miles in 50 minutes run around the park
★ Not too short to scribble frenetically as I write in my diary
★ And not too short to fiddle regularly

No. But they are too short to do the one thing I have spent the last three days attempting to do: fist myself. Since Ben did the three-finger slide on me, I have been curious to find out what it might feel like to have a whole hand inside me.

So I have been stretching, contorting and bending until I'm doubled over, and I still can't get my fist in past the knuckles. I'm sure I could fit my whole hand in – but I seem to be hindered by the length of my arms and they just won't reach far enough to give me the 'angle of perfection' that I am looking for. Dammit!

Is it possible that I cannot fist myself? Maybe I'm just going to have to rely on a willing lover to do it for me instead.

I do hope I can find someone who will oblige.

Friday 25th March

'You know what I really need?' I said to Fiona, as I took a swig from my Martini and looked at my phone beeping with another text from Blog Boy. 'I need something easy and simple with a guy; none of this "I like you, but the timing is wrong" stuff – it's too much hassle.'

Fiona nodded at me. 'Don't we all, darling; that's the problem – it's always complicated. Men – they're just not able to do things without getting their knickers in a twist. They're just as fucked up as we are, probably more so.' She pointed at my phone. 'Still calling you, eh?'

I nodded. 'He said he just wants to be friends ...'

'And you? What do you want?'

I shrugged. 'Well, I'd love to shag him; that goes without saying. But, I like him as a person too. So, I don't know ...'

'Let me ask you a question, then,' Fiona said, finishing off her mojito in a quick gulp. 'If he called you tomorrow and said he was keen on getting to know you, what would you say?'

I thought for a moment. 'OK, you got me: I would probably say yes, but I would also want to shag him as soon as I could.'

Fiona laughed, 'Of course.' Then she looked at me seriously. 'But he said he didn't want to get involved, didn't he?'

I nodded.

'Look, Abby, forget him. Don't bother; it's just wasting your time. Find someone else – a bloke you can just shag – have some fun.' She winked at me. 'What about him over there?'

I turned and saw a lanky blond guy drinking a pint at the bar. Fiona certainly knew my type: he was gorgeous, but barely into his twenties.

'I think he's a bit young,' I said, and turned back to her.

'They're always grateful for an older woman's experience!' Fiona replied, and we both laughed and carried on chatting.

Later, as we staggered drunkenly to our separate bus stops, I saw the young guy again. He appeared to be waiting for the same bus as me.

What luck, I thought, this must surely be fate.

As the bus pulled in, the young guy got in the queue behind me.

'About time the bus arrived!' he said and grinned at me.

Bless. Young and sweet. How cute. I smiled back at him.

We made small talk, found empty seats and sat next to each other. It turned out that he lived down the road from me, and again I felt as though fate was trying to tell me something: shag this young man. So I flirted with him. And when we got off at the same bus stop, I smiled at him, moved towards him and kissed him softly on the lips.

He hesitated for a moment, slightly shocked by how upfront I was, then leaned in and snogged me back. It wasn't long before his cock was pressed up against my thigh and I was whispering in his ear that he should come back to my place and fuck me hard.

He didn't need me to ask twice; he grabbed my hand and we made our way up to my tiny flat and fell drunkenly onto my bed.

We shagged with a gleeful passion and he was certainly enthusiastic. Ten minutes later and he was ready to go again, but the fact that he was ever ready didn't make up for his lack of technique. I think he must never have done anything other than fuck like a rabbit – and I don't mean the battery-operated version, either.

All he was capable of was the old in-out, in-out pump action, and in my drunken state I couldn't be bothered to intervene and teach him a thing or two. If it hadn't been a one-night stand I would have shown him some new tactics but three (self-inflicted) orgasms in, I just wanted to roll over and go to sleep.

When we woke up this morning, he told me he was 22 – ten years younger than me! I suppose that explains everything. It was only after I'd packed him off home that it occurred to me that he might have been a virgin. Hope to God I didn't scar him for life, but when I remember the grin on his face as he hammered away, I don't think that's likely.

Could have just been his surprise at scoring at the bus stop, though.

Tuesday 29th March

'Franklin is a lovely guy,' Kathy said to me last night, as we polished off the meal she had just cooked.

'He sounds it,' I replied, gulping down some more wine and beginning to feel it going to my head.

'It's such a shame. He's been in a state for a while now.'

'So it wasn't amicable, then?'

Kathy shook her head. 'God no. She was a complete bitch to him. They haven't spoken for months.'

'Poor bloke. He's been taking it badly, I imagine?'

'Well, they were together for over a decade. And now they hate each other.'

'Fuck, that's horrible. I can't begin to imagine what he must be going through now.'

'Well, his self-esteem has taken a hit, but he's doing a bit better now.'

'Good for him.'

'But you know what Franklin really needs?' Kathy asked, as she poured me another glass of wine.

'A shag, I bet. Lots of meaningless shags.'

'Yup. He hasn't been single for a very long time, you know – not since his early twenties. He's probably got no confidence with women at all now.'

'Fuck, he missed out on the mid-twenties shagging around thing, then?' I remarked, sad on his behalf.

'Exactly; she was the only person he slept with that whole time. And now he's got a lot of catching up to do.'

'Poor bloke. I feel for him.'

'He's very cute, you know,' Kathy said, as she took a large swig of wine from her glass.

'I'm sure he is,' I said, gulping more wine down too.

'You'd like him,' Kathy grinned at me slyly.

'He sounds like a decent chap.'

'You two would get on brilliantly, he'd have you laughing all night.'

'Kathy, where are you going with this?'

'I think you know.'

'You want me to shag him, don't you?'

'Oh, come on! It'd be a win/win situation!'

'Not necessarily true.'

'Why not?'

'Well, for starters, he's just come out of a long-term relationship.'

'And therefore he's in need of some fun. I know you would make sure he had that.'

'Well yes, but no. You underestimate where his head might be at. He's hurting right now – having a shag might just screw with his mind, rather than help him.'

'OK, true, but I also know that he's not looking for anything meaningful, so a quick shag might give him the boost he needs to feel happier about himself,' Kathy said, trying to sound persuasive.

'Well, fair enough,' I agreed, 'in terms of ego-boosting. But I still think it's dodgy: a one-night stand with a girl he picks up in a bar is probably a better idea.'

'But he's been out of the game for more than a decade. What makes you think that he would even be able to chat up a girl?'

'Fair point; but the fact that he knows you and I know you, would put him in an awkward situation, don't you think?'

'Not at all. The very fact that I know you both means that neither of you are random fuckwits. He would relax with you more, I think, than with some stranger.'

I shook my head. 'I disagree.'

'Why? You're a nice person, relaxed, laid-back, friendly. You wouldn't take the piss out of him, or take advantage of him, and you are good in bed. Well, you sound like you are, anyway.'

'All true, cheers! But you are forgetting one very important factor.'

'What's that then?'

'He's only slept with one person over the last decade.'

'And?'

'And,' I continued, 'faced with another woman, he might feel anxious …'

'I doubt it,' Kathy said, unconvinced.

'Hear me out …'

'OK …'

'He might worry that he won't be able to satisfy her. How can he know that the skills he has used on the same woman over the last ten years will transfer to another woman so easily?'

Kathy pondered on this for a moment.

I continued, 'And even though he may be totally wrong, with that in mind, he may end up losing his erection, or coming too quickly, or, even not at all.'

'True. But knowing you, you'd just end up doing something else and still having fun, right?'

'Yeah, of course; it's no big deal to me, whatsoever. But for him, it'd be a different story. He may feel embarrassed about it, and because we both have you as a mutual friend, it may worry him that his "prowess" – or lack of – gets "reported" back to you.'

'I see what you mean,' Kathy said, nodding.

'What I am saying is, if he were to go soft with a stranger he picked up in a bar, he might not give a shit, because he would never have to see them again. But being with me, and knowing me, through you, is a different matter.'

'I agree with what you are saying – really. But I still think he would be up for it. He'd like you, I know it. And you two could have some fun together.'

'How do you know he'd even fancy me?'

'Come on, what's there not to fancy? You're intelligent, sexy and have big tits. He's into buxom women big time.'

'Well, that's a starting point I suppose, but who's to say that five minutes into a conversation with him, I don't find him yawningly dull and he doesn't find me brain-numbingly boring?'

'Oh, for fucks' sake, Abby. I know both of you, you'll get on like a house on fire, trust me.'

'OK, OK, enough said, but honestly though, he's not looking for anything serious right now, is he? Because I don't want to go there if he is.'

Kathy laughed. 'No, not at all. You'd be like a bit of light relief to him, helping him move on.'

I frowned at her. 'You make it sound like Franklin is a charity case.'

'He is. Come on, he's gorgeous, funny, sexy and broken-hearted. And you need a shag. How can you say no?'

'I'm not sure about this.'

'Oh, come on! Think about it, OK?'

'Alright. I'll think about it …' I said, and meant it.

The Girl's Guide to Date Speak

What is said	Women mean	Men mean
I'll call you in the morning to confirm our lunch	Before 11 a.m.	When you're just about to buy a sandwich, I'll call
I'll call you in the afternoon to confirm our dinner	Before 4 p.m.	Just as you're heading out the door to meet me for dinner
I'll call you later	Later today	Possibly at some point in the future
I'll call you tomorrow	Tomorrow	Maybe in the next few days; maybe not
I'll call you at the weekend	Between Friday and Sunday	Sunday or Monday – after the football
I'll call you in a couple of days	2–3 days	4–6 days
I'll call you in a couple of weeks	Within 2–3 weeks	Possibly within a month or so
I'll call you soon	Within a month	I'll keep your phone number handy just in case we meet again
I'll call you sometime	I'll keep your phone phone number handy just in case we meet again	I'm about to delete your number from my phone
I'll call you	Please call me	I will never call you

4

April

Monday 4th April

When I read back over my diary for March it struck me that every time I had sex, I had a multiple orgasm. It's just seems to be a given now, though I remember when it wasn't always so. Like many women, I went through a period in my life when I found it difficult to climax. Back in my early twenties when I was in a relationship with a man called Rupert, I almost never had an orgasm. If I masturbated it was no problem, but during intercourse, nothing. It all ran like clockwork. A bit of fumbling foreplay, then he entered me, thrust a few times and ejaculated. By the time he had finished I was just getting started, but that was the end of my chance of coming. Instead I would lie there while he snored, wondering how it was that *he* got all the fun and *I* got *none*.

I suspected that it had something to do with the fact that he always came moments after penetration, and that our timing was totally mismatched, but I found it stupidly difficult to be open about this with him without hurting his feelings and making things even worse. I didn't want him to go soft if I said something like, 'Er, would you mind holding on a bit so I can come?'

Alternatively I could ask for more foreplay, but he wasn't so great with his hands or mouth, so that was ruled out. I needed to think of a way of postponing the inevitable, so that I could have a chance to be stimulated enough to climax. Eventually I hit on the best solution: perhaps if I made him *think* that before he gave me his cock I had to be begging for it, then it would give me a chance to get aroused before penetration and thus asssist with me obtaining an orgasm.

I flirted with the idea one night:

Me *(licking his cock lightly)*: 'You want to know what *really* turns me on?'

Him *(grinding his hips into my face)*: 'Mmm, what?'

Me: 'Well, you know how much I like your cock? How I *love* feeling it inside me?'

Him *(his cock rubbing against my lips)*: 'Yeah, I love it too, you feel fantastic.'

Me *(swirling my tongue along the shaft)*: 'Well, because I like it so much, because it turns me on *so* much, I want you *not* to give it to me.'

Him *(his cock bouncing along my tongue)*: 'You want me *not* to give it to you?'

Me *(sucking the tip)*: 'Yes. Don't give it to me. It'll drive me *crazy.*'

Him *(grabbing his cock and whacking it against the side of my face)*: 'I'm not sure if I get you. How do you mean?'

Me *(nibbling the head)*: 'I want you to *withhold* giving me your cock. Don't let me have it. It'll drive me nuts.'

Him *(paying attention now)*: 'Really?'

Me *(squeezing his cock tightly in my fist)*: 'Yes. I'll be *begging* for it, if you won't let me have it.'

Him *(gleeful)*: 'Mmm, begging, I like the sound of that.'

Me *(sliding my hand along the shaft)*: 'Yes, even if I beg, you *mustn't* let me have it.'

Him *(getting excited)*: 'Yeah. I won't give it to you, not even if you cry for it.'

Me *(both hands on his cock now)*: 'Yes, but if I beg and beg and plead and cry, you'll give it to me eventually, yes?'

Him: 'Hmm. I *might* ...'

And low and behold, it worked.

When we were next in bed, instead of ramming his cock into me at the first opportunity, or fumbling around with bad foreplay, he stayed fully clothed and refused to let me play with him at all. I couldn't have hoped for better: I got to dry-hump him for ages. It was the perfect non-direct clitoral stimulation I needed to finally give me an orgasm prior to penetration and make me wet enough for it when it happened.

Our excitement was synchronised for the first time, and when he eventually 'gave in' to my 'demands', the three minutes of penetrative sex that he was capable of brought me off too. We climaxed together for the first time that night.

And I learned that to get what I want in sex, I should always make suggestions to my partner when I had his cock in my mouth. A very valuable life lesson I think.

Wednesday 6th April

Fiona and I met up in a bar near Oxford Street tonight, ostensibly to catch up with each other, but really just to ogle some talent. There weren't really many nice-looking guys in the bar though, mostly middle-aged bankers, so Fiona and I ended up chatting for most of the evening.

At one point I was queuing for the loo when a sweet-looking blonde girl approached me. I was expecting her to ask me if I had any tampons, but instead, she asked me something really odd:

'Are you looking for a friend?' she said, in a thick East European accent.

Confused, I asked her to repeat the question. She whispered again, conspiratorially:

'Are you looking for a friend?' and beamed at me.

For a brief moment, I wondered to myself, is she offering me her *services*? I've read about prostitutes soliciting for customers in bars, but surely not in a toilet? Especially not the ladies'. I feigned ignorance, 'I'm sorry? I didn't catch that?' She motioned to one of the cubicles and said:

'There's a girl in there. Are you looking for a friend?' and then she smiled at me again and lightly touched my arm.

This was a new twist, was she *pimping* someone else? I let out a resounding 'No!' and acted shocked and a little disgusted. Her smile faded. She pointed at the stall door again and said quietly, 'There's a girl in there crying. I wondered if she was your friend. I didn't know what to say to her. I hope she's OK.'

My cheeks burned with embarrassment and I muttered something intelligible and locked myself in another cubicle, hoping that the toilet would swallow up some of my stupidity. By the time I crawled out she was nowhere to be seen. I made my way back to Fiona and told her the whole story, which she thought was hilarious.

'Anyway,' Fiona said, much later, when we had ingested far more wine, 'if you're so worried about girls, why not try one out – see what they're like?' She put her hand on my knee and winked at me.

I know not to take Fiona seriously, however playful she

gets with me, because I know she's just a flirt by nature, but she had a point. I wanted to try new things, so why shouldn't sleeping with a girl count? Fiona could help me too, as she had plenty of experience in such matters. I told her she was right, and then we started our ogling again, but this time I was checking out the women as well as the men.

We both noticed a beautiful girl dancing near our table. She was truly striking: slim, curvaceous, with a sumptuous arse over which she was wearing a body-hugging wrap dress and absolutely no underwear. I looked *many* times for a panty-line and couldn't find one. I couldn't stop staring at her bum; it was like a siren, calling 'squeeze me, slap me'.

Fiona saw me looking and removed herself by sashaying off to the loo, 'If I were you, I'd take this opportunity to approach her.' And lo and behold, I didn't need to budge an inch. The beautiful girl immediately came over to me, sat next to me, put her hand on my thigh and flicked her hair back coyly, then firmly demanded that I come and dance with her. Nervous, I teased her back gently, but stayed seated. I wasn't brave enough to dance with another woman in public, even though, dammit, she was lovely, and sure enough my pants were moistening already.

By the time Fiona came back from the toilet, my would-be seducer had given up on me and gone back to dancing with her friends. Fiona called me a chicken and I knew she was right, but if I'm only just getting used to chatting up men, I'm in no position to try to pick up a woman. Yet.

I think I need to make it my next objective, though. This is one thing I have to experience – even if it will take all my confidence to do it.

Diary of a Sex Fiend

Thursday 7th April

I'm still shopping around for men and adventure but now I'm doing it on-line. Internet personals. I didn't know where to start, but Tim recommended Craig's List and he was spot on – it's the funniest thing I've read since Blog Boy's diary posts.

I wonder which of the following got the most responses. This one?

'*Ladies, this really is quite straightforward. If you are in need of some oral stimulation, send me a message. No shagging or blow job required in return. The only condition is that you are not a "minger".*'

Or this stupendous promise?

'*If we hit it off let me take you back to my hotel to give you multiple orgasms through oral and good hard sex*'.

Or this modest offer?

'*We are two good-looking guys looking to fulfil the fantasy of having no-strings-attached sex with one woman. We are both well endowed and have already had a threesome with one girl. We are looking for someone who will take double penetration and two in one hole. You must be prepared to be awake for at least seven hours as we both have huge amounts of stamina. Our last conquest didn't sleep all night and came about 25 times.*'

Or you could even buy-one-get-one-free with this generous guy:

'*If you like the idea of a cute guy pulling out his hard cock and wanking it until he shoots, then get in touch. The thrill's in the performing, but I'm happy to lend you a hand, too, if you wish.*'

And here's some wishful thinking:

'*I want sex, so mail please, this afternoon would be good! nice fit birds with pics, please.*'

If this is all that's out there, I think I need some other options ...

Saturday 9th April

Tim took me to an R&B event in central London this evening. I was half hoping we might both get lucky, and I did, but not in the way I was expecting.

We were dancing away to some hip-hop and I noticed this woman near me. She was an angel, a stunning smile, almond eyes, long black hair flowing down to her fantastic arse and a cleavage to die for. Gorgeous.

But, you know, it was a straight club, she was a girl and I was nervous, so I turned away from her and carried on dancing with Tim.

Tim went to fetch some drinks and I sat down to rest my weary feet. Stilettos *are* every bit as painful as they look, and the balls of my feet were burning. Unbelievably, the Angel suddenly reappeared and sat down next to me in the booth. She plunged straight into a conversation with me so easily that I guessed she must be drunk or on something else altogether, and I found myself intimidated, but chatting back.

Her body language was uninhibited too, and she wasted no time resting a hand on my knee. Wow. I could barely move. She kept up a stream of talk and laughter, then eased her hand up my thigh, and I didn't object, but was fascinated by the confidence she radiated.

At some point, Tim came back and I introduced her to him, then she grabbed my hand and told me to follow her. I grinned stupidly at Tim as she pulled me across the dance floor to the women's toilets. She led me into a cubicle and sat down on the lid of the loo for a cigarette. I stood over her, and we both laughed like this was the most natural thing in the world for two women who'd only just met. Then she grabbed me, pulled me down and kissed me.

My mind was reeling, trying to work out what the hell was going on, 'Ah yes, this is what I'm doing. I'm kissing a girl in the toilets in a club. And not just any club, a straight R&B club, possibly the most homophobic environment you'll get. And I'm the only white girl in here, and am I gonna get my arse kicked when I get out of here? And what will Tim think? And God, her tongue feels so fucking delicious in my mouth …'

I just went with it. I straddled her and she kissed my neck while I stroked her shoulders. She put one hand on each cheek of my bum and tried to hoik me towards her, but we couldn't get close enough and had to stand up against the cubicle wall. She pressed against me, her thigh between my legs, and I shoved mine between hers. I felt our breasts touching, and even her nipples hardening against mine. It was totally intoxicating, and I could barely breathe when she caressed my breasts and the sensation seemed to run right through my entire body.

She peeled my top off, unhooked my bra and brought both her hands to my tits, cupping them in her fingers. I did the same with her, struggling for a second with the clasps behind her back before freeing her amazing boobs, and then we rubbed breasts together, skin against skin.

I wanted to take it further, right there and then, but we were rudely interrupted by her friends who banged on the door and demanded that she come out. We dressed rapidly in silence and she unlocked the door, making some excuse to her mates about 'having a smoke'.

I immediately went to find Tim, who was pissed off with me for disappearing, but when I told him about my girl-on-girl action he cheered up immediately and demanded to know all the gory details.

Typical bloke.

Tuesday 12th April

My encounter with the R&B angel made me question a lot of things. It was very enjoyable, but still, I can't help thinking that given the choice I'd rather have a cock between my legs than another woman's thigh, no matter how sexy.

I find it funny when men I know joke that if they had breasts, they'd be fondling them all day. If some good fairy granted me a cock I would never, ever leave the house, my hand would be so glued to it (quite literally after a while, I imagine).

I do find penises extraordinary. To have this thing, this part of your body, that you can see *grow* with desire, watching it change from a flaccid state to one of pulsing hardness fascinates me. Plus you can see how aroused you are without the aid of a mirror.

It must be hard though (again, quite literally) to have the focus of your sexual being physically hanging outside your body. If a bloke got turned on as many times a day as I do, he'd be fighting off erections all day – rather inconvenient in the workplace. There are definitely advantages to women's evolutionary make-up because I'm not sure how many people would be willing to fight for a man's right to have erections in public. Well, apart from me, of course.

There are other bonuses to having a cock (not to mention the ability to command higher wages), but the one I would be most interested in – the one I wish I could experience – would be the ability to slide it inside a woman and feel her climax around it. I would have loved to have been able to do that in the R&B club on Saturday night.

When it comes to women's bodies, I'm sure that I think about them like any straight man. If I see a beautiful woman I'll find myself looking at her breasts and imagining them in my mouth, I'll look at the curve of her arse and think how gorgeous it would feel gripped by my hands, and I'll look at the dip between her legs and wonder what she would feel like there if she was soaking wet.

I want to be able to:

★ Stand behind a woman, lift her skirt, tease her breasts and slide a cock into her
★ Lie side by side and rub her clit before slowly pushing a penis into her
★ Grasp her ankles and enter her with a slow and shallow pace until she is begging to be pummelled

Which is basically everything I like to have done to me by a bloke.

Using my fingers wouldn't be enough though, which is the problem. If I were a man I'd be able to penetrate her with a part of my body that was my own sexual nerve centre too. And that's something.

So, with apologies to my lesbian sisters, no finger, however skilled, is a substitute for a hot, swollen cock. Not that I'd turn down another rendezvous with the Angel or any other beautiful woman, it's just that I'd be more inclined to go for it if I knew I was going to get a thorough *dicking* at the end of the night, too.

Thursday 14th April

On the internet again last night, I ended up in some chat rooms, instant messaging with a man. I'm intrigued by the way people take on different identities on-line. The barriers are down too, paradoxically, but that makes it easier by far to chat someone up.

Him: 'You have a great arse. Can you send me another picture? It's getting me hot!'

Me: 'It's much nicer in the flesh, I guarantee it!'

Him: 'What are you doing right now?'

Me: 'Apart from sliding my fingers between my legs and imagining your cock?'

Him: 'Meet me.'

Me: 'What?'

Him: 'Let's meet.'

Me: 'We barely know each other.'

Him: 'Which makes it even more fun. Meet me. For a drink. We can go somewhere brightly lit and public if you're worried.'

Me *(trying to think seriously for a moment, but being distracted by the throbbing between my legs)*: 'OK, then. Café Bohème, Soho; one hour.'

Him: 'Don't be late!'

I wasn't.

I lucked out. He was much more dashing in person than

on the web, his greying sideburns highlighting an easy-going smile. We drank a couple of glasses of wine and flirted, his hand never leaving my knee. It wasn't long before we were kissing, my pants still soaking from our internet chat earlier.

I was dying to fuck him – I'd been horny all day, wanking all afternoon and now I was sucking face with this man who had made all my will power fly out the window. I needed to bed him – and fast.

I thought about my options:

1) Go back to his = unsafe. He could be a psycho, despite appearances;
2) Go back to mine = unsafe. I don't want him to know where I live in case he's a stalker;
3) Go to a hotel = too expensive;
4) Go to a friend's place = too embarrassing;
5) Fuck in the bar's toilets = cramped.

Sod it, I thought, cramped it is.

So without further ado, I seized his hand from my knee, pulled him down the stairs and pushed him into a cubicle in the ladies' loos. I unzipped him to find him rock hard already, and got on my knees to suck him deeply.

'Aargh! Fuck!' he pushed my mouth away. 'That feels too good – I don't want to come yet!'

I grinned at him and he pulled me up to kiss me, sliding his fingers between my legs and round the gusset of my knickers. With his lips crushed into mine I came almost immediately, shuddering against him. Breaking away for a second, I groped for a condom in my purse and rolled it onto him. Standing up? No. Me on his lap? No – the toilet was too narrow.

'Turn around,' he said hoarsely, and pushed my hands up against the back wall. I leaned over the cistern and braced myself. With barely inches to spare in the cubicle, he entered me from behind and thrust as much as was possible – which wasn't much.

It didn't take long – he was way too worked up – but it was fun while it lasted.

Even though I forgot to ask what his name was.

Sunday 17th April

Things I recall about last night:
★ Eating a lovely meal cooked by Franklin
★ Laughing as I spilt red wine on my top
★ Making a joke about using my tongue to scoop out the inside of a Creme egg
★ Drinking glass after glass of red wine
★ Downing two double shots of absinthe
★ Playing footsie under the table with Franklin
★ Seeing Kathy and her boyfriend smoking cigarettes in the garden through the living room window, as Franklin sat there, hard cock in his hand and said to me, 'Suck my cock. Please. Suck it. Now.'
★ Kathy and her boyfriend going to bed
★ Franklin and I knocking everything off the kitchen table as we kissed
★ Us moving to the couch
★ His fingers inside me
★ Me climaxing
★ Putting a condom on him

★ Him fucking me from behind

★ Me running to the bathroom to vomit violently

★ His fingers in my arse

★ Me climaxing again

★ Me attempting to put a condom on him, but he already had one on

★ Him fucking me up the arse

★ Me begging him to 'fuck me harder' as I held onto the arms of the couch

★ Me climaxing again – hard

★ Waking up with the sunlight burning my eyelids and him smiling at me

★ Having the most intense, pulverising, agonising pain in my head

★ Rubbing my hands over his cock as I tried to get him to slip it in between my legs

★ Falling asleep again

★ Upon waking, telling him that I felt I had to explain why I'd had anal sex with him:

    a) Because I had only done it with Steven before

    b) That I was in love with Steven at the time and therefore it was a special, intimate thing for me

    c) That I had only done it a couple of times

    d) That I was amazed that the alcohol had made me so enthusiastic about Franklin doing it

    e) That I was going to write about it in my diary, to try to understand why I had done something so intimate with someone I hardly knew

Things I don't recall:
* How I got all the bruises on my arms and legs
* Whether or not I sucked Franklin's cock at the table
* Taking off my own or his clothes, but leaving my stockings on
* Sucking his cock
* Playing with his cock
* Him licking me
* What he felt like inside me
* Whether he climaxed
* How many times this happened and when I blacked out
* How long we had sex for

Things I regret:
* Drinking so much. Never again will I:
  a) Drink one and a half bottles of red wine
  b) Drink two doubles of absinthe
  c) Mix wine and absinthe
* Not remembering the events of the night
* Not knowing whether he climaxed
* Doing something as intimate as anal with someone I had no feelings for
* Shagging him under the influence
* Ruining Kathy's lovely white tablecloth with red wine

Things I am pleased about:
* That my worries about Franklin not being able to get it up were totally wrong. Which is nice for him.

Diary of a Sex Fiend

Thursday 21st April

I've been away the last few days, having a quick break with Fiona down at her mum's flat in Devon. It's been wonderful.

* ★ The sun shone
* ★ The air was fresh
* ★ The green hills were lush
* ★ And the orgasm I had whilst sitting in the middle of a field was a real mindblower

Not that it was premeditated. I just wanted to go for a refreshing walk to clear my head and breathe in some oxygen after all that London grime. The last thing on my mind was outdoor masturbation in broad daylight.

It all started off so well. I strolled lazily along the beach, sinking into the soft sand and getting an eyeful of the rolling waves. I climbed the dunes and surveyed the surroundings: green hills behind me, the ocean in front of me, clear blue skies above. I turned away from the sea and followed a little path that led between the fields and discovered a bench on it with a view of some charming thatched cottages in one direction and the dunes and the bay beyond it in the other ...

The sun beat down on me and the wind ruffled my hair and I could hear the sound of a buzzard overhead looking for prey. It was heavenly. I felt relaxed. I felt calm. I felt ... horny.

I tried to ignore it, hoping it would go away if I focussed on the view rather than the pulse between my legs. No luck. All I saw was sex: when I looked at the fields, I imagined sitting on top of a guy, riding him, our nakedness contrasting with the lush greenness; when I looked at the ocean, I imagined being shoulder deep in the water, my legs wrapped around a guy's hips, his cock plunging into me; when I looked at the sand dunes, I imagined a guy standing before me, his jeans undone, me on my knees, his dick in my mouth.

I sat there on my bench and my pussy throbbed. Something had to be done – and fast. I unzipped my jeans, slid my hand between my legs, and – not caring who could see me on this little country lane – frigged myself into oblivion. A minute later I had an explosive climax.

Job done I sat back and watched nature carrying on its business: the buzzard gave up the hunt and disappeared into the distance, the waves kept on pounding the shore, the sun went on shining. I felt blessed. I felt alive. There's nothing like an alfresco wank in a beauty spot – call it getting in touch with Mother Nature.

Monday 25th April

Three things I really must remember the next time I go jogging in my local park:

1) Take three Ibruprofen at least an hour before exercising because having painful period cramps during a run is no fun. (Note, I continued on regardless, such is my dedication to having sculpted muscular thighs.)
2) Make sure iPod batteries are fully charged before leaving the house. Halfway into the run you need music, not 20 minutes with silent headphones just when fatigue is kicking in. It's somehow more difficult to run without The Departure blaring in my ears.

3) Ensure all randiness is dealt with prior to leaving the house. It's annoying to require a fiddle while running at speed across an open space. (And no, there was not going to be any more outdoors daylight frigging: it's one thing to be masturbating on a country lane in the middle of nowhere; it's an entirely different matter doing it in a London park.)

N.B. At least I always go for a wee first. I'm no Paula Radcliffe. I am a lady.

Friday 29th April

Met up with Blog Boy this evening. It was the first time we'd seen each other since he asked to keep things strictly platonic. I knew when I made the date that it was going to be tough, and I was right. I spent most of the evening trying not to fancy him. The problem is that he has presented so many good qualities for inspection so far:

★ Good-looking guy – check
★ Intelligent – check
★ Funny – check
★ Thoughtful – check
★ Interesting – check
★ Fun to be with – check
★ Tall – check
★ Sexy – check
★ Large hands – check
★ Good kisser – double check

It's like a switch has been flicked in my brain, and now I *can't* see him as just a friend. That's all he wants though, so I have no choice but to try to relate to him on that level.

When we chatted over dinner tonight, it took all of my concentration to focus on NOT staring dreamily into his eyes; it was a struggle for me NOT to touch his hand as I laughed at his jokes; and it took all my resolve NOT to peek at the blond fuzz (or at least, not a second time) curling out of the top of his shirt and think about running my fingers through it …

When we said goodbye to each other and I leaned in to peck him goodnight on the cheek, I had to muster all my strength to stop myself moving my lips closer to his and kissing him properly.

But I did it. And he did too. We both behaved well – as friends, you might say – and I'm hoping that we can continue to build on this and develop a really good friendship now. I think he's a top bloke and I look forward to getting to know him some more.

Though I shan't be telling him that I keep trying to imagine what he looks like naked. At least, not yet.

The Girl's Top Ten Guide to Chatting Someone Up

1 Get visual of subject in sight. Try not to drool over their sexiness

2 Check for wedding ring on finger; then check for tan-line of removed ring. If nothing's there, you are free to go ahead. Unless they use a tanning salon, in which case you're screwed

3 Smile at them; don't grimace: you are being friendly, not showing off expensive dental treatment

4 Give direct eye contact. Try not to stare. Or to let your eyes wander over their crotch/breasts

5 Introduce yourself, offer your hand out and shake theirs with confidence. Do not give a bone-crushing grip, or a wet-fish. Be firm and friendly

6 Find out about the other person, ask them questions. People are essentially arrogant and love to talk about themselves: use this to your advantage and feign interest if necessary – they'll find you even more attractive if you listen well

7 Build a rapport. I recommend the two-tier method:
a) Verbal: agree with them as much as possible.[1] The key is making them feel that you have something in common with them, even if it is just empathy[2]

---

1. Obviously this does not apply if they are a) a Tory, b) a sexist pig, c) are so boring that they can only talk about shoes, shopping or football.
2. Do not, however, pretend you are less intelligent than them, or that you are only interested in getting in their pants (even if it is true).

b) Physical: not in the first instance, sexual.[3] Use body language – mirror their movements and behaviour. If your body matches theirs, unconsciously they will feel more attracted to you.

8 Once rapport is built, and some time has passed, drop the question. I recommend something similar to the following: 'I hope I'm not being too forward here; I was wondering if you would like to go out for a drink with me sometime?'

9 Be prepared for one of the following responses:
a) They laugh at or ignore you
b) They run away
c) They smile awkwardly and then make an excuse and leave hurriedly
d) They say 'Thank you, I would love to say "yes", and if I was single I definitely would.'
e) They say 'Thank you, that would be lovely, when did you have in mind?'

10 If it was a 'no' do not allow any embarrassment you might feel to get the better of you. Although rejected, and shag/meaningful encounter-less, at least you put yourself out there, and took a risk: life is too short to let opportunities pass you by. Plus, you boosted someone's ego and made them feel good, which is always a nice thing to do. Even if they do suspect that you went home and wanked about them later

---

3. Touching their private parts comes later, when you know what the score is.

5

May

Sunday 1st May

Franklin sounded subdued when he called: 'I thought you would have phoned me by now.'

I hesitated. 'Sorry. I wanted to.' *But didn't want to give you the wrong idea.*

'You wanted to?'

'Yeah. But I felt kinda weird after being so drunk.' *I delayed calling you because I was worried that you might be too into it.*

'So, you regret that night, then?'

'No, no, not at all. It was great.' *What I could remember anyway, but I do regret drinking so much and feeling like I was out of control. I scared myself doing anal with you: it was something sacred and special that I shared with Steven. Doing it with you made me miss him.*

'So you really don't remember much?'

'Not really, but I do remember enjoying myself. A lot.' *I wish I could recall what your cock looked and felt like; what a tragic waste to have been too drunk to remember.*

'I had fun too, but I remember everything.'

'Really? Would you mind answering me some questions then?' *Oh God, this is going to sound so offensive.*

'Go ahead.'

'Um. Right. When we sat at the kitchen table and the others were across the room, you had your cock in your hand, yeah?' *I remember how much that turned me on; you telling me to 'Suck it.'*

'Yup.'

'Did I suck it?' *If I did I am such a slut.*

'You most certainly did.'

'Wow.' *I am such a slut.*

'You leaned over the table and gave me some fucking great head, actually.'

'Oh, thanks.' *Jesus, Kathy was ten feet away and I was sucking a penis at her dining room table. How uncivilised of me.*

'It was lovely.'

'Did we have sex for long?' *I remember throwing up, passing out and having three orgasms, but not what your cock felt like inside me.*

'A couple of hours, I guess. You really don't remember, do you?'

'Sadly no. Um, look I have to ask you, did you come?' *I remember our using condoms; I don't recall you pumping yourself into me.*

'Ha ha, yes, twice. You were fucking hot, I can tell you. You really fucking turned me on.'

'Thanks. I'm glad to hear you had fun too.' *Thank fuck for that, I was feeling very guilty that I was the only one pleasured that night.*

'Fun? Abby, let me tell you, doing anal with you was fucking amazing, I had a lot of fun.'

'It was great for me too.' *It scared me how much I begged you to do it.*

'Actually, Abby, I feel honoured that I was your second. Especially now that I know that it's a special thing for you.'

'Thanks.' *My head has been in a mess trying to figure out how I could do something like that with someone I have no feelings for.*

'You were my first actually.'

'Your first? I thought you said you'd done it before? You certainly seemed experienced in it.' *There's no way my arse could have been fucked like that by an anal virgin.*

'Not in anal.'

'What then?' *Oh dear, I think I know.*

'You were my first since the break-up.'

'Oh. I didn't know. I'm sorry.' *Liar.*

'Yeah, it was a big deal for me, actually.'

'Really? I didn't know that.' *Liar liar pants on fire.*

'My head was all messed up after that night, I suppose it is fair to say.'

'I bet. It must have been tough for you.' *Oh fuck. I didn't want to be the rebound one. Fuck.*

'And I thought we had got on really well. So I was confused when I didn't hear from you.'

'We did get on well. We had lots of fun. I didn't contact you straight away because I am in a weird place right now and I am not sure what I want.' *I didn't call you because when we woke up, you smiled at me, and pulled me close, and stroked my hair. And when you looked in my eyes, I saw a longing that terrified me. You were so affectionate and caring and loving and it all felt wrong after knowing you for less than 24 hours. And it reminded me of what it is that I want and I felt hollow and empty inside knowing that I didn't want this with you. I don't want to be the replacement for your ex, just because you are hurting; I can't be. I had to make sure you weren't going to get attached to me, so I was letting some time pass until I felt it was safe to call.*

'Me too. I am all mixed up. Not sure what I am doing right now.'

'So listen, it doesn't need to be a bad thing. We had a good time, right? We get on well. We don't need to be a head-fuck for each other when we can have a laugh instead.' *If you weren't freshly out of a long-term relationship and heartbroken, I would consider you as Potential Boyfriend Material, but for my own emotional safety I am making sure you remain a good-natured one-night stand. Though I wouldn't mind having another go, sober.*

'Yeah. Perhaps we could meet up next week, or something?'

'OK, let's speak then.' *If only you could be a fuck-buddy, then it would be fine, but when you're pining for her, fucking me is only going to hurt us both.*

'And I feel honoured you let me fuck you up the arse; it was truly magnificent.'

'Ta, luv. It was pretty damn great for me too.' *Though my arse cheeks were sore for two days afterwards.*

Thursday 5th May

How to be political:

★ Wear an ironic protest-vote 'Backing Blair' t-shirt. Combine with a denim mini-skirt, black hold-up stockings and leather ankle boots with a four-inch heel.

★ Be aware that random strangers will stop you in the street/park/pub and ask you questions about the general election.

★ Make sure that you have prepared your arguments about the benefits of a hung Parliament or a small Labour majority. Be ready to challenge the myth about the Tories getting in.

★ Ask how the other person is going to vote. Be enthused about protesting and explain the concept clearly.

★ Ignore them looking at your tits/legs/arse, even if they're fanciable.

★ See that you are winning them over to your side. Have confidence that your argument has possibly inspired one more person to get out and vote.

★ Carry on walking down the street/jogging in the park/drinking beers at the pub and know that you have done your little bit for democracy.

★ Stay up to 5 a.m. seeing the results come in.

★ Watch the Labour Party win, but with a massively reduced majority.

★ Go to bed and have a celebratory fiddle.

Thursday 12th May

There's a handsome man lying in the grass in my front garden. He is fully dressed. And drunk.

I did debate for a moment whether it would be in his best interest to snog me, seeing as he's such an attractive chap and obviously in need of a good woman to look after him.

Then I considered taking advantage of his situation and removing some of his clothing to get a peek at the goods.

And then I wondered whether I should call an ambulance for him – he is very inebriated, after all.

Instead, I decided I should help him manoeuvre himself into the recovery position so that I'd at least know that he was safe, even if he did pass out. I don't think I'll invite him in, in case he pukes all over my house, but if he's still there in the morning, perhaps I'll invite him in for a coffee.

Tuesday 17th May

Met up with Blog Boy again last night. We went to a cast and crew preview screening of a film I worked on last year and I think he was a little impressed that we had to go to BAFTA to watch it. Unfortunately the film itself wasn't likely to score a BAFTA, it was actually laughable in places, which was a shame.

Still, it was fun to see it with Blog Boy. Our knees and arms were touching for the entire duration of the film. I know I shouldn't read anything into it, but I'm positive there was something there between us.

And I'm sure that it wasn't just the heat emanating from between my legs.

Sunday 22nd May

A few days ago I got talking to a journalist that I'd met through Fiona, and she mentioned that one of her colleagues was writing a piece on anonymous sex. His task: to find a woman who was willing to turn up and fuck him with no strings attached.

Naturally I was excited by this prospect; here was a chance for me to have some casual sex and skip the whole drama of meeting, chatting and getting to know someone. Forget on-line assignations, here I could just turn up, have a shag and leave, and this bloke would write about it and never even know my name. I wouldn't have to go to the trouble of finding out his, either.

It sounded intriguing, so I suggested to Fiona's friend that she pass on my email address to him, and if he was interested, he should get in touch.

He emailed just an hour later. He seemed like a nice enough guy, sincere, and Fiona's friend vouched for him, so I knew he wasn't some hind of pyscho. So today was the day that we arranged for me to go to his house and fuck him.

I was nervous, of course, partly through fear that we wouldn't fancy each other, and partly because I'd never done anything as remotely daring as this before, but I set out to Ladbroke Grove well armed: see-through basque, black stockings, tiny g-string, knee-high boots, condoms and lube. Let's just say I like to come prepared.

I rang the buzzer and he opened the door almost immediately, and we grinned at each other a bit stupidly then kissed quickly on the lips. There was a spark though, thank God, and I followed him upstairs to his bedroom, getting an eyeful of his shapely backside as we went.

It started off well. We kissed some more, clothing was removed. I went down on my knees and sucked his cock. He put a condom on, pushed me onto my front, slipped his cock into me and began to fuck me from behind. I was so excited that I came straight away. He took my hips in his hands and pushed himself in deeper and I climaxed again, bucking against him.

Then he fucked me more vigorously, and I shuddered so much that I pushed his cock out. He tried to penetrate me again, but his penis had gone soft. He sat down on the bed and proceeded to tell me that I reminded him of his ex and that he was too upset to shag any more. Then he rolled himself up in his duvet and turned away from me.

No matter how horny, how sexy, how hot the moment was, there was nothing like the passion-killer of the ex being brought to the bed too; we lay there for an hour or so talking about how broken-hearted he was – not exactly the aphrodisiac I wanted in this type of situation.

I did wonder what I was doing there, listening to some guy I didn't know pour his heart out to me about another woman, when he should have been giving me a good rogering. But I felt bad for him. Being with me just reminded him of how much he still wanted and missed her, and I'm not such a bitch as to take my pleasure and leave. He deserved to be treated with respect and given dignity, even if I found the whole affair sad and pretty annoying.

Besides, I'd had three orgasms to his none, so I felt it only polite to listen to him.

Wednesday 25th May

Between them, the journalist and Franklin have given me plenty of food for thought. I've considered some other men I've slept with too and come to the conclusion that a lot of men are crap at one-night stands. The thing is, they want intimacy, but can't accept that and seek solace through casual sex instead, only to find that that's inevitably unfulfilling for them.

The idea that men use love to get sex and women use sex to get love must be a myth. In my experience men want and need love and companionship *just as much* as their female counterparts and women seek sexual pleasure and gratification *just as much* as men do.

The difference is that it's still largely unacceptable for men to admit to that emotional need in case they are labelled 'weak' or 'feminine', and if a woman is open about her sexual desires she's instantly a 'slut'. So we don't question the gender stereotype and it's no surprise that this internal emotional frustration can be a source of conflict between the sexes.

I reckon that this suppression of feelings is the root of men's insecurities and that this eventually manifests itself during bedroom antics: going soft or coming too quickly seems common for many men during casual sex. As a result, I believe men fall into one of three categories:

1) **The Fucker**. They are immersed in an existential emotional crisis, about which they are in complete denial. They seek to fuck as many women as possible as a way to feel better about themselves.

   The sex they have is cold, distant, emotionally detached, and purely masturbatory: they use the woman's body to get off – her pleasure is irrelevant.

2) **The Pseudo-Partner**. They either haven't had much casual sex or have recently come out of a meaningful relationship. They seek a connection with a woman and convince themselves that they just want a shag but are actually seeking emotional solace, either to boost their damaged ego or because they miss that shared closeness with someone.

   The sex they have is very affectionate, loving and tactile: they interact with the woman as if she were a partner.

3) **The Lover**. They may be newly single or just want more casual interactions on their way to finding that someone whom they connect with emotionally. They are not necessarily seeking sex just for the physical pleasure, but are open to all opportunities that cross their paths – even if that might mean ending up in a relationship with someone who was originally just a one-night stand.

   The sex they have is generous, fun and laid-back; they interact with the woman as if she were a friend, enjoying her intellect as well as her body in bed.

I seem to have met quite a few Fuckers in my time; they're responsible for the *horrendous* interlude that was my early twenties. I had sex with men that not only didn't give a shit about me, but actually *pretended* to give a shit about me in order to get me into bed. They told me that they had feelings for me and wanted to see me, but *never* contacted me again.

Sex with these men was dreadful, without exception. They fucked me as if they were the only ones with sexual needs and that all that mattered was their cock. I felt used, unsatisfied and empty, just a means for them to obtain their pleasure.

Being emotionally fucked up, these men kept lying to themselves about 'just wanting a shag', spent all their time lying to women in order to have awful, selfish sex, and then went about their lives in denial. I bet they left a lot of messed-up women in their wake.

Sex with a Pseudo-Partner is much better in terms of quality, but comes with its own baggage, this time at the other end of the scale. These men are unfamiliar with the necessity to keep a degree of emotional distance during a one-night stand and they resort to making love instead, even though they'll swear blind that they only wanted to get laid.

They don't want just physical gratification, but crave affection which they end up expressing sexually with someone they don't really have feelings for – it's a false intimacy, in every respect.

I've read about Pseudo-Partners time and again on sexblogs, and it looks like a lot of them end up seeking solace in the arms of a prostitute who offers a so-called 'Girlfriend Experience'. They get sex, a cuddle and a chance to offload what's on their mind instead of the clock-watching in-out, in-out that usually constitutes an appointment with a working girl. These men can then pretend to themselves that they are getting what they want – even if it is just for one hour. And by paying for it, it helps to maintain the charade that all they want is a shag.

Keeping up these appearances can be tiresome, however, and it seems to be quite common for men to have difficulty sustaining an erection when faced with casual sex. The journalist may have *thought* and *said* that he wanted a quick shag, but his flaccid penis was telling a different story – and a cock never lies.

I'm not saying that bedding a Pseudo-Partner can't be enjoyable – the journalist was a great lay, which I'm sure was because he had had plenty of practice with his partner – but in a one-night stand situation, his lovemaking became ultimately unsatisfactory. I wanted to be fucked with abandon, and he wanted to snuggle up and lie in my arms.

It's not all doom and gloom, though, because I've saved the best for last: The Lover.

Tom is a great example of this type of man. He is emotionally aware, upfront about what he wants and open-minded about what he might encounter.

His expectations do not seem to be centred round his need to suppress his emotions, nor does he suppress his sexual desire; rather he is able to have creative, laid-back sex if that is what he feels like having, or something more deeply felt if he prefers.

There is *nothing* soul-searching or angsty about the things he does – he has always told me honestly what he wanted from me and I have done likewise with him. The sex was flirtatious, spontaneous, tactile and relaxed. The true physical expression of sexual desire got explored and the experience was mutually enjoyable, and, of course, sexually satisfying on multiple levels – quite literally.

A Lover like Tom understands the difference between making love and fucking: he may shag with abandon, but he can still do it in a generous and sensual way, without resorting to that false intimacy and make-believe lovemaking.

Tom can also cut through the crap: if he wants to see me again, he says so, if he doesn't, he'd say that too, I'm sure. He is mature enough to relate to me as an equal and as a friend – even if he's fucking me senseless. Challenging the myth about them just wanting sex, men like Tom are able to connect on an intellectual and emotional level too; unlike the Fuckers or Pseudo-Partners, there's no game-playing, so The Lovers make great one-night stands.

Sadly for me, Tom has ended up getting back together with his ex-girlfriend in Birmingham so that rules out future commitment-free romps and I am left *still* looking for men who don't make the aftermath of a casual shag messy, complicated, uncomfortable or embarrassing.

I've hardly come across any Lovers so I suppose that proves my hypothesis. How depressing. Still, I maintain my optimistic outlook. I have to, after all; if I didn't I'd never get laid, and right now I am gagging for some more action.

The Girl's Top Ten Guide to One-Night Stands – for Women

1 Be clean, hygienic and keep your muff neat.

2 Wear nice pants. Clean ones are a must. Especially if you are planning on draping them over someone's face at some point during the night

3 Always take condoms with you. Practise putting them on a dildo with your hands and also with your mouth: the latter skill especially helps when they go soft at the sight of a little bit of latex

4 Relax for goodness sake: it is just sex. It doesn't need to mean anything

5 Enjoy it. Sex is supposed to be fun, not stressful. Don't spend time focussing on your insecurities:

a) If you are getting naked with him, know that he fancies you and you turn him on

b) He doesn't think you look fat; if you feel confident about your body, he won't notice the cellulite

c) Don't worry about not being porn-star sexy: if you are enjoying yourself, that will make his cock hard – not your trying to seem at ease with maintaining a fantasy representation of women

6 Enthusiasm is more important than experience. Do ask what he likes, and whether he is enjoying what you are doing; always be willing to learn new things – even if they are not to your liking (anything involving defecation, children or animals obviously doesn't apply here)

7 Don't worry if you find it difficult to climax. Instead of feeling pressurised to come, concentrate instead on that nice warm feeling in your pussy and enjoy it. If all else fails, move his hand away and do it yourself. Mama knows best, remember

8 Do try to remember his name. Though you could probably get away with 'God', 'Jesus', 'Ah yeah, fuck me harder' and 'Do it! Do it!' if you are unable to recall who you got into bed with. He won't mind

9 Don't be too affectionate, loving or tactile, nor expect him to be: this is casual sex, not a relationship

10 Make sure you understand the etiquette after the event:

a) If he says: 'I'll call you' and walks out – he means: 'Goodbye'

b) If he says: 'That was great, thank you. Want to do it again sometime' and gives you his phone number – he means: 'I'd like to shag you again'

c) If he says: 'That was great, thank you. I had a wonderful time – and not just because the sex was fabulous; the company was terrific too. If you'd be into meeting up for dinner sometime, give me a call' – he means: 'I'd like to see you again and get to know you some more'

d) If he says: 'We are made for each other' – run

e) If the sex was fantastic, but you don't want anything more, even though he might, it could be tempting to use the guy as an occasional human dildo; but be aware of hurting his feelings if you decide to do so (unless he behaved like a total tosser, in which case, ride his cock till it makes you come, and then get the fuck out of there)

The Girl's Top Ten Guide to One-Night Stands – for Men

1 Be prepared: hygiene and cleanliness are *not* optional here – especially in the trouser department

2 Pant choice can be important - always go for the newest ones you have, and *obviously* they should be clean. Style is not that relevant; though it takes a confident man to get away with wearing y-fronts

3 Always have condoms handy; there are *no* excuses here. Brand type is irrelevant, just ensure they are nearby as the moment 'arises'. Do try to stay hard – it helps

4 Relax for goodness sake: it is just sex. It doesn't need to mean anything

5 *Enjoy* it. Sex is supposed to be fun, not stressful. A one-night stand is not a job interview: it's about having fun, not about your sexual prowess

6 Enthusiasm is more important than experience. Being willing to learn and be open-minded will make for much better sex than attempting to be the world's greatest lover

7 Don't worry if you lose your erection. It's really not a cause for concern – sex does not depend on your ability to stay hard – just be willing to do other things to please her and yourself. Whatever you do, *don't* say 'Sorry, honey, it (pointing at your cock) ain't happening tonight' and then roll over and go to sleep. *Do* slide your fingers inside her, kiss her deeply and say, 'God it turns me on to see you so worked up, I could do this all night' and then *prove* it

8 Do try to remember her name rather than just call her 'honey', 'darling' or 'babe'. Obviously don't call her by the wrong name, or worse, 'Mother'.

9 Don't be too affectionate, loving or tactile; this is casual sex, not a relationship:

a) Making love is reserved for partners, not one-night stands

b) Intimacy can confuse the situation

c) If you want a 'Girlfriend Experience', go hire a prostitute

10 Make sure your etiquette after the event is up to standard:

a) If you say: 'I'll call you' and don't mean it – you're a tosser

b) If you say: 'That was great, thank you. Want to do it again sometime?' and hand over your phone number – you might just get a call for another shag

c) If you say: 'That was great, thank you. I had a wonderful time – and not just because the sex was fabulous; the company was terrific too. If you'd be into meeting up for dinner sometime, give me a call.' – do make sure you give her your phone number too, or else you'll look a right twat.

6

June

Wednesday 1st June

'You know what you were telling me about that guy you shagged and how him getting all emotional frustrated you?' Tim said, somewhat cautiously.

'Yes,' I answered. 'What about him?'

'Well, I've got an idea about how you can avoid all that business and still have some fun …' I could practically hear Tim grinning down the phone.

'Do tell.'

'There's this place – a nudist spa – where people go and … you know …' he trailed off.

I was confused. 'No. What?'

'They, um, well … It's a swingers' place. Where people go to have group sex. We could go – if you like.'

There was silence for a moment. The word 'swinger' echoed round my brain. I had heard the term of course, but I always associated it with the images from the TV show 'Eurotrash' where fat middle-aged people greased themselves up in oil and made home videos of each other. Not really an appealing thought.

I couldn't deny that my curiosity was stoked, though, and after the disaster with the journalist, I was eager to try something new.

'Tell me more,' I said, still wary about what was coming next.

I heard him take a deep breath, 'Look, I went to this place a couple of weeks ago; it's somewhere couples go and have sex with strangers – other couples – and everyone is cool and they're all our age. I've been waiting for the right moment to mention it to you. I thought maybe now would be a good time for you to try it. We don't need to actually do anything if you don't want to, but it would be fun to watch, don't you think?'

I pondered on this for a moment. It was certainly a good suggestion, but there was one problem: we weren't going out with each other.

'It sounds interesting, Tim, but how would we fit in? We're not together and, please take this the right way, as much as I like you I don't really want to shag you. You're my friend and I'd like to keep it that way.'

'No, no, no, we wouldn't have to shag!' Tim exclaimed. 'We could just go there together and if you wanted to try anything, you'd know that I'd be there to support you. And, um, if you didn't mind me being around I could just sit in a chair and watch – making sure you were safe and everything.'

I laughed. '*Safe*, eh? Like you don't get off on watching – I know you, Tim!'

He laughed too. 'Yeah, OK, I wouldn't say no to being a voyeur, it's true. But seriously, if you're up for going, I would be there for you, not for me. I just want you to see this place – it's amazing.'

'Let me think about it, OK?' I said, half making my mind up there and then.

'No pressure,' Tim replied, 'But I guarantee it'll be an adventure if we do go.'

'Let's hope,' I said, and began to fantasise about what it might be like, knowing full well that my curiosity had already gotten the better of me.

Saturday 4th June

Dear God,

I know we don't have a close relationship, and that's something to do with the fact that I am an atheist and I don't believe in you, but putting that fact aside for a moment, I'd like to have a little chat.

You see, I have a bone to pick with you. It's not about the tsunami that devastated so many lives six months ago. Nor is it about the fact that millions of people are afflicted by HIV and AIDS as a result of following the Vatican's mindless dogma. It is not even about the way that huge parts of this planet are dying due to needless waste and selfishness on the part of its participants. No, it is about a much more important issue: I think I have become a sex fiend.

Although I do not hold you directly responsible for the issues that arise as a result of my condition, it is, I think, fair to say, that you are interfering in at least part of the process. Since it appears that you 'move in mysterious ways', I can only assume that you have some connection with my own particular cycle of events.

An example:

I am not a fan of the police force. This might be because I once spent 11 hours in casualty after getting my head cracked open by a particularly sadistic copper after presenting myself as a 'threat' when I sat down in the middle of a street on a non-violent demo. Even when I have handed out flowers to riot police as a peace offering, I have still been beaten by their truncheons and riot shields.

In my opinion, put a riot uniform on any copper and you get someone hungry for power and prone to vicious outbursts. Most policemen seem not to be the most progressive of 'new' men – racism, sexism and conservatism are all endemic within the force. I don't believe the 'it's only one bad apple in the barrel' view: in my opinion, they're all representative of a pretty nasty section of society.

So, dear God, it came as something of a surprise to me today when I found myself lusting after a copper. In all honesty, God, I am rather annoyed by it and I want a full explanation from the responsible parties, ie, you.

There I was minding my own business, buying my copy of the *Guardian* in the newsagent's, looking forward to a hectic day of sunbathing, coffee and reading up on current events. I didn't expect to be witness to a violent dispute between my neighbours, and I certainly didn't expect to be checking out a policeman's arse and wondering what his body was like under his uniform.

It began innocuously enough. A van full of police arrived, separated the brawling parties and began to take statements from everyone. My interviewer just happened to be a rather handsome thirty-something well-built man, with lively blue eyes and dark blond hair. Not that I was paying attention to his looks or anything. It was just an observation – I am *very* perceptive about such things.

He asked me lots of mundane questions, and apologised for the dullness of them, trying to crack some jokes to liven things up. I found myself answering him sarcastically, and he chuckled as I took the piss when he couldn't transcribe my answers fast enough.

As we chatted about what had happened and joked about my dumb neighbours, I suddenly twigged that not only was I laughing out loud at this policeman's jokes, but I was twirling my hair between my fingers and stroking the back of my neck. God, I was flirting with him.

When he walked over to his colleagues to check some details, I became aware that I was scoping out the wonderful curvature of his delightful bottom, too. As he conferred with them I glanced down and saw how erect my nipples had become – they were poking through the flimsy t-shirt I had quickly thrown over my bikini top like bullets. Shit, I was turned on as well.

He came back over to me and we continued chatting, and I attempted to will my nipples into a state of relaxed submission. I don't think it worked, since his eyes darted over them more than a few times. Then I noticed his chest. His shirt was open just enough for me to idly imagine undoing the rest of the buttons and running my fingers through his hair, finding his nipples and caressing them gently. I tried not to mentally undress him any further, but it was no use: as he stood there and flirted with me, he was as good as naked in my mind's eye, his cock as hard as the truncheon on his belt.

Dammit. He was a copper. A fascist in uniform. A power-hungry Servant Of The State. Why was I attracted to him? Why was I wondering what it would be like to kiss him? Why was I imagining ripping off his navy blue trousers and running my fingers around his balls?

Something is wrong – very wrong in my world. All I can think, God, is that, in your mysterious way of doing things, this must be part of some larger Plan of which I'm unaware. I'm sure that you have a Reason for this to happen and that your Will manifested itself in this insane attraction. It certainly can't be explained any other way. I may be a sex fiend, but I can categorically state that I will never shag a member of an organisation that's seen fit to club me over the head in the past. Even if he *is* devilishly handsome, with a cute smile and a fantastic arse.

So, with this in mind, I would like an explanation. You know, some kind of sign to give me an insight into these events. You don't need to do anything flash like a thunderbolt or a storm, but sending me the winning lottery ticket or even a new gorgeous man would certainly help me understand things a little better. I like to think it would put all the disturbing recent happenings into context and restore my rational perspective on the world.

Waiting to hear from you, on my knees as always,
Abby

Tuesday 7th June

Got an odd text from Blog Boy. I'm sure he's flirting with me. Not that I have anything against that, but surely 'just friends' means sexual innuendo should be avoided?

Especially since with me, it tends to lead to other things.

Sunday 12th June

When Tim and I arrived at the spa in Willesden last night, I was very nervous, even though I had downed two double whiskies to try to take the edge off my anxiety. I could see scores of people walking around in towels, and several who were just stark naked.

I don't have an issue with nakedness, but being a nicely brought-up English girl and accustomed to British prudishness, it did seem odd to be able to see so many breasts and penises on open display.

But I soon got over it.

I suppose it helped that Tim almost immediately whipped off his clothes and strutted his stuff.

Nice arse, I caught myself thinking as I checked out his physique, faintly remembering how I squeezed it tightly when we fucked each other many years back.

I was a little more self-conscious than Tim, though, and I tucked the complimentary towel I was handed on entry to the spa as tightly as I could round my breasts before joining him for a stroll around the place.

The ground floor had a handful of jacuzzis, a couple of steam rooms, a small swimming pool and a sauna, plus plenty of communal showers. I noticed a flight of stairs leading to another floor.

'What's up there?' I asked Tim.

He grinned at me. 'Wait till later; I'll show you then.'

My interest piqued, we settled down into some lounge chairs opposite a spa pool and watched the place begin to fill up with people.

I was surprised how many young twenty-something couples were there, blending in with the thirty-something crowd who were in the majority; I had thought Tim and I might be the youngest – I was wrong. Everywhere I looked were handsome guys and fit girls; things were certainly looking up.

After a while, Tim coaxed me to join him in a jacuzzi, then leapt in bollock-naked, leaving me on the edge feeling like a twit and still clutching the towel. I had to take the plunge at some point, so I threw it off and stepped into the warm water, noticing everyone eyeing my body as I did so, making me self-conscious.

There were four other couples in the water with us, all naked too. Tim and I just sat there and smiled cheesily; everyone else was more talkative.

After a few minutes' cooking in the overheated water, I noticed two of the couples getting very friendly, the girls laughing out loud together. Suddenly they began kissing, their partners egging them on. Tim quickly shot me a knowing look: I told you so.

I beamed at him and then stared, along with everyone else, as the girls shifted so that they could each straddle their own partners whilst continuing to snog.

I began to throb between my legs as I saw the guys reach out to their partners and fondle their tits; I couldn't believe what I was seeing. Before I knew it, the two couples had become a mish-mash of hands, mouths and breasts, the girls rubbing themselves against the guys whilst they kissed passionately. God, it was hot.

Then one of the girls pulled back, whispering in the other girl's ear as she smiled at her. They both nodded to each other, and with that they stood up and began to get out of the jacuzzi, with the guys following – their erect cocks at full mast.

I couldn't help but stare. Tim pulled me out of my daze, saying softly, 'Let's follow them; I want to show you what happens next.'

Stunned, I got out of the water with him, grabbing my

towel and his hand and we made our way up the flight of stairs I had seen earlier. We just caught sight of the two couples from the jacuzzi disappearing into a small room off a central hallway.

I could see there were lots of doors leading off the hallway – at least five or six. The door of the room the two couples had gone into was firmly shut, however. I was a little disappointed – I was very curious about what might be going on behind that door.

'This is where it happens,' Tim said, and gestured down the hallway at all the doors.

'What happens?' I asked, half knowing how he would answer.

'The playing,' he whispered. 'If we hang here, we may get to see something – often they leave the door open for people to watch, or join in.'

I nodded, as if this was the most normal thing to do in all the world: stand in a hallway in a nudist spa and wait for couples to have sex so that we might watch them.

I was filled with fear at the prospect, yet I was also transfixed. The thought that I might get to see some real live action was enough to stop me from fleeing into the night in total embarrassment. Tim held my hand protectively, and let me know that I was safe.

We didn't have to wait long. We heard some noises at the end of the corridor and quietly made our way to a small room, poking our heads round the door.

I couldn't believe what I saw.

On top of a wide bunk was a girl on her knees getting fucked by a guy doggy-style. In front of her, a bloke was shoving a cock into her mouth. To her side was a man busily jerking himself off.

They all looked up as Tim and I peeked into the room. My heart raced and I felt myself blush.

'Join us!' said the guy getting a blow job. 'Come in.'

I looked at Tim and he saw the terror in my face.

'Thanks, we're just going to watch – if that's OK,' Tim said, and I suddenly felt reassured: he was looking out for me.

The girl stopped sucking cock for a minute and turned to look at me. 'You're cute,' she said and grinned. 'Are you sure you don't want to play?' She gave the penis in front of her a little lick and its owner groaned loudly.

I giggled nervously. 'No, thank you. I am a voyeur tonight, and it looks like you have everything in hand.'

She smiled at me and then resumed what she was doing, the men carried on merrily too.

Tim and I stood there for a while. We watched her climax and then climax again, and the guy stroking himself exploded all over her back. All the while I was aware of the thud-thud pulsing between my legs, as I watched and heard the passion in the room.

Tim touched my arm and hissed, 'Let's have a look around – there's more to see. I think you're going to like it.'

I nodded and we left the foursome to continue their antics.

Tim led me to another set of stairs and gestured that we should go up.

'What's this?' I asked, slightly apprehensive again.

'This,' he said somewhat proudly, 'is where the action *really* happens.'

I must have looked petrified, because he put his arm round me, 'You're going to like it, I promise.' And with that, he led me up the stairs.

The first thing I noticed was the heat: it spilled down the

stairwell and as we approached the open-plan room it hit me full in the face. I could smell sex in the air and as I brushed my hand against a wall to steady myself in the darkness, I found it was dripping with moisture. The air was literally thick with passion.

We let our eyes adjust to the dim light and as shapes began to take focus, I scanned the room for detail.

Four couches filled the space, each with two or three naked couples sitting on them. In the centre of the room, two couples were straddling each other on the floor.

At first I couldn't make out what they were doing, but it soon became clear.

I could see four or five hand jobs, three blow jobs, two guys eating pussy, two couples fucking cowgirl-style, two couples fucking doggy-style and two couples on one couch all playing with each other – the boys and girls changing partners from time to time.

I couldn't help but stare. Thank God it was so dark in there, my eyes were on stalks.

So this is what swinging is all about then. Now I get it. Now I understand. The couples get off on watching – and being watched – by other couples. I began to hear – and see – orgasm after orgasm and I felt myself getting even wetter. I wondered what it would feel like to be part of the mass of bodies surrounding me.

Tim fetched me out of my erotic daydream. 'Here, let's sit,' he said and motioned to a spot next to one of the couches.

I looked at him in confusion – why move? He nodded behind me, and I saw a group of guys, dicks in hand, watching the action. Quickly, I joined him on the floor, not wanting to spoil their view or their wank.

We sat there for some time and just gazed. I don't think I have ever seen – or heard or smelt for that matter – anything as sexy as what I could see before me. I was drenched.

Tim leaned over to me and whispered in my ear. 'Was I right? Do you like it?'

'I love it,' I said. 'It's so fucking erotic. Wow.'

He grinned at me. 'Is it turning you on?' he asked and then whispered even more softly in my ear. 'Is it making you wet?'

My pussy tingled as he spoke and a part of me just wanted to lean over him, slide my hands around his penis and fuck him hard, but I knew it wasn't a good idea. As if he read my mind, Tim said, 'I've got a fucking boner; wish I could do something about it, but with us being friends and all, it'd be a bad idea.' He shrugged and I nodded in response.

'Anyway,' he continued, 'I brought you here to see what it's like; we can both go and wank ourselves silly on our own later – we shouldn't complicate things by acting on impulse now.' Again, I nodded and was pleased that he could show that restraint. I, on the other hand, just wanted a cock in me and could barely think straight for all my horniness.

I tried to focus and turned to watch a youngish, stunning couple who were busy shagging in front of us.

It was wonderful to watch two people be so free with their sexuality; sharing their pleasure in front of others. As the guy fucked his girlfriend from behind he caught me staring at him and beamed at me. I smiled back and as he fixed his eyes on mine, he pumped her harder. She began to climax and he winked at me. I suddenly felt part of his pleasure – of their pleasure – and I found myself wondering what it might be like, were I to experience that close up rather than from afar.

But I was getting frustrated. With Tim there I couldn't

even play with myself, let alone him. Swinging must be great, but only if you've got someone to shag, that is.

Worn out with horniness, I suggested we leave and Tim and I made our way downstairs to get dressed. After I exited the changing room, the guy who winked at me suddenly approached me, his girlfriend on his arm, both of them looking spent and friendly.

He handed me their phone number and said they would love to entertain me this weekend and would I call them if I was interested?

My heart raced with excitement and I smiled, saying yes I would.

And I think I just might.

Wednesday 15th June

Blog Boy rang tonight. We talked about his work getting in the way and laughed as innuendo somehow seeped into our conversation.

I know the fact that we talked about sex doesn't mean anything – I'd be stupid to think it did – but I can't help but wonder if maybe he is getting second thoughts about the whole 'friends' thing.

The way we are flirting right now makes me think that maybe something will happen with him – even though he is going abroad soon.

I guess if he did want to test the water and date me, I wouldn't say no.

Certainly not if a shag with him was on the cards.

Diary of a Sex Fiend

Thursday 16th June

I finally plucked up the courage to ring Ellie and Will, the good-looking couple from the nudist spa. I don't know why I was so nervous: they took turns on the phone, chatting to me in a friendly way, and immediately put me at ease – there weren't any awkward silences during the conversation.

I suppose I initially felt a bit odd because it's not every day that you phone someone to make a plan to have your first threesome. But after our half-hour flirty talk, I feel much more relaxed about the whole idea and we have now arranged for me to visit them tomorrow evening.

I can't wait.

Friday 17th June

Ellie picked me up in her car and we drove to Will's flat in Barnet. How appropriate, I thought, going to suburbia for a hot night of swinging.

It was Ellie's idea for us to meet up beforehand; she said she wanted to put me at ease and that there was no pressure to do anything because this night was about having fun and getting to know one another.

But, she added, if we were to all end up in bed together, she wanted to establish some ground rules first. We discussed the basics: safe sex, full consent, no pain, likes and dislikes. It all seemed pretty straightforward. I was going to have sex with Ellie and her boyfriend. Yippee – my first threesome!

However, it turned out it wasn't as simple as that. As we

pulled into the driveway on the estate, Ellie mentioned that she had one main rule for the evening.

'What's that?' I asked, thinking that she might say 'no photographs' or something like that.

'You're not allowed to fuck Will,' Ellie replied. 'You can do anything else, but penetration with him is exclusive to me.' She put her hand on my knee and smiled.

Oh great. The one thing that I enjoy and now it's off the menu – fabulous. How helpful that she waited till we got here to tell me that. If she had mentioned it before, I might have been able to bail out. Now I am stuck, committed to a three-some where I don't get fucked.

I looked at Ellie for a moment. Her top was open and I could see her cleavage poking through it. My pussy responded to the sight.

Fuck it, I thought. I'm not going to get any cock tonight, but at least I can finally learn what it is like to go all the way with a woman.

I put my hand on Ellie's knee and she leaned in to kiss me. The night had begun.

It didn't take long for things to really get underway; two bottles of wine in and Ellie was flirting with me on the couch while Will looked on eagerly.

Ellie and I started to kiss again and she quickly pulled off my top and started stroking my boobs.

'God, that's so hot,' Will murmured. 'You both look beautiful.'

I grinned at him and wondered if he was getting an erection. I was certainly wet.

I removed Ellie's top too and we rubbed our tits together. It felt lovely. We started tugging off the rest of our clothing and beckoned to Will to join us. He didn't waste any time stripping off, and, cock sticking out like a flagpole, slid his arms around both our waists and kissed us each alternately.

It felt delicious. The contrast of his rough face against my lips and then her smooth one was divine; I wanted to fuck them both simultaneously.

After a while, Will pulled back. 'I want to watch you both,' he said, his hand slowly stroking his cock.

Ellie and I obliged. We lay on the sofa cushions and kissed and stroked each other, her fingers pushing between my wet thighs, mine between hers.

So, this is what it is like to finger a girl, I thought, as I felt her wetness and circled her clit slowly. She moaned and I slipped a finger inside her, shocked by the heat of her. She rocked against me and I pushed another finger inside as she gasped in delight.

Will was getting more and more excited; he'd alternate between stroking my breasts, kissing Ellie and then switching back. It felt lovely.

Except for one thing. She was crap at fingering.

I suppose I had expected that, being a girl, she would know what to do, but I soon realised that sharing the same physiological make-up is irrelevant when it comes to sexual skills. Ellie fingered me as if she was polishing an ornament and trying to rub out a tough stain. It hurt, and was pretty unpleasant.

I was trying to be polite though – I was, after all, being given the opportunity to shag two people at once. I should be nice about it. So I didn't ask her to adapt her technique but just flinched and dried up and wondered how much longer I could hold out for.

Thankfully Will took over; his deftness immediately brought me close to an orgasm. I would have climaxed too, if it were not for Ellie suddenly saying she was uncomfortable with him fondling me and that she wanted him to stop.

Oh great. So I'm on the verge of finally getting off and now she doesn't want him fingering me. I thought it was just his cock off the cards? Now it's his hands too?

I felt robbed, but yet again I didn't say anything. It seemed inappropriate somehow.

When Ellie got down on her knees and suggested I join her sucking Will's penis, I relaxed again – at least I was going to get some cock action tonight.

So we sucked and lapped and licked and kissed together and it was good again; I felt connected to them both, involved and very turned on.

After a while, Will pushed us both onto our knees in front of him and we presented our arses side by side. I heard Ellie gasp and looked back to see Will sliding his dick into her. At the same time, he slid three fingers into me and for a moment, he fucked both of us; one with his cock, the other with his hand. We all moaned together.

But when Ellie then noticed that Will had his fingers inside me, she suddenly jumped up and stormed off. Will removed his hand and went after her, licking his fingers as he did so and shooting me a sly look, whispering to me 'You taste beautiful,' as he left the room.

I lay there, unfulfilled and frustrated and attempted to wank to relieve myself.

I could hear them arguing next door: Ellie accusing Will of crossing their boundaries, him defensively saying that his cock had gone nowhere near me. They shouted for a while and then I heard her crying. Finally Will came back into the room and I, somewhat guiltily, stopped playing with myself.

'Ellie's a bit upset,' he explained. 'She's gone to bed. I'm going to join her.'

I nodded and shrugged.

'Sorry about things,' Will said. 'I guess we thought we were ready to do this, and we weren't.'

I tried to smile and not think about Will's cock and how horny I still felt. All I needed was a quick rub …

'Look,' Will said, 'If you're ever up for it in the future, you know our number. Do give us a call.'

'Sure thing,' I said, lying.

Will grinned and then kissed me on the lips. 'See you in the morning,' he said, leaving me alone in the living room.

I lay there and tried to refocus on the task at hand: giving myself some release. A few minutes later, after a hot thought involving Blog Boy's tongue lapping at me, I was done.

But I couldn't sleep; my mind was too busy.

I waited for daylight to arrive and when it did I got dressed, grabbed my things and left.

I spent the time thinking about what had happened as I waited for the first tube home. It all seemed to have gone horribly wrong. It has certainly made me think twice about what it might be like if I was in a relationship and we dabbled in a threesome.

I thought that the group thing was supposed to be easy? I guess I am learning that it is a lot more complicated than it appears.

Especially when feelings are involved.

Sunday 19th June

After the threesome with Ellie and Will turned sour, I've been revisited by memories of some other awful sexual encounters. Thankfully, most of them aren't recent.

Years ago I slept with a man who was dreadful in bed. He was beautiful, and I assumed wrongly that his bedroom skills would be as glorious as his looks, but my opinion proved totally misplaced.

I was 18 at the time, naïve and sexually inexperienced but curious. I was working in TV, mingling with the 'rich', 'famous' and seemingly 'glamorous'. I enjoyed my social life and the attention I got from men. I was hungry for new experiences.

So when this outgoing, funny, drop-dead gorgeous man from Los Angeles joined our department for a short time, I eyed him up with some interest. Not that I was the only one; I noticed how all the women preened themselves when he walked into the room, flirting with him and laughing outrageously at his jokes. Here was a fantastically sexy, charming man, and he was single. Every woman was out to bed him.

Not me though. He was 36. I figured he would never be interested in a young girl like me. In my naïveté and ignorance, I truly never thought he would be interested in me because of this very fact.

So, when he flirted with me, I just took it as friendly work banter and thought nothing of it, and when he asked if I would show him round the city, it just seemed like an innocent request, albeit one that flattered me immensely.

It only struck me that he was attracted to me after the arm he'd placed round my shoulder in the dark of the cinema slowly travelled down my neck and began fondling my breast. A cheesy move for a teenager, let alone someone 18 years my senior, but it felt nice, so I didn't complain. When his hand wandered down my back and ended up caressing my arse, I didn't stop him doing that either. It was only when his fingers slid in between my butt cheeks and began rubbing against the crotch of my tights that I pulled his hand away. I felt embarrassed, self-conscious, dirty. We were in public after all.

But I liked what he had been doing. Even with my inexperience, I knew how aroused he had made me, so when he suggested going somewhere private, I agreed, and we left the cinema pronto.

We ended up at his friends' house in a beautiful bedroom complete with a four-poster bed, white drapes over the huge floor-to-ceiling windows, and candles on the oak floor. A recipe for romance, one would think. Wrong.

It all started off well: sensual kissing, some gentle breast play, but as if he'd suddenly pressed his foot down on the accelerator, he went from stroking me one moment to ramming his fingers in and out of me as hard and fast as he could the next. I wasn't even wet. It hurt and I tried to get him to slow down, but he just fumbled and tried to push his fingers inside me again, and I got more and more turned off.

Looking back, I am a little surprised at how bad he was. I mean, not only was he 36 and surely should have known better, but when I tried to guide him and show him what I liked and how he could turn me on (and, obviously, get me wet enough for his cock to fuck me), he just wasn't interested. It was as if he had a preconceived idea about what sex between us should be like and he wasn't going to alter his plans no matter what, even if that meant I didn't enjoy myself at all. Of course I was too amateurish myself then to either insist on a different course of action, or to try to switch the attention onto him, so that his heavy-handedness wasn't so apparent.

After much fumbling he put a condom on and attempted to enter me. It was pretty obvious it wasn't going in; I was as dry as a bone at this point and the last thing that I wanted was a big cock forcefully rammed into me with no lubrication.

So, my pussy shut its doors and put up its 'Closed' sign: no entry to you, mate. He did try – for most of the night – but to no avail. No more sex was had, though he begged me to stick my tongue into his arsehole and jerk him off with my hands. He called it 'tromboning'. I am pleased to say I politely declined: I am a good, clean English girl – the very thought!

In the morning we left for work together, but agreed to enter the office separately, so that people 'wouldn't talk'. We carried on our jobs as normal, no one guessed anything, and we barely spoke again. I didn't feel any animosity towards him, but something more like pity, I suppose. When the other women in the office were drooling over him I just shut my mouth and kept quiet. No need to ruin their fantasies, or destroy his reputation or ego.

But thinking about it now, especially after Steven's infidelity with a much younger woman, I understand how ignorant I was about the whole affair. Here was a man, twice my age, who tried to pressurise me into having sex when I didn't want to.

What an arsehole.

Diary of a Sex Fiend

Monday 20th June

Kathy's boyfriend keeps looking at my breasts. Granted, they aren't small bosoms, but he blatantly checks out my tits in front of her, and it's really troubling me.

The thing is, I know that men look. That all men look. But surely they should do it surreptitiously and not in front of their potential/future wife's eyes? His eyeballs, however, seem permanently locked onto my tits and he fixates on them whenever he is in the room with me, regardless of whether she's there or not.

I can't understand why he's so obvious, given that:

1) I'm Kathy's close friend;
2) Her boobs are bigger than mine;
3) We might both notice him looking.

It seems odd that he would take the risk of being found out by staring so blatantly. I'm sure Kathy knows he is looking, and if she doesn't, that she would be thoroughly pissed off if she spotted him.

Without trying to blow my own trumpet, I'm not ruling out the possibility that maybe I represent some fantasy material for them both, and that not only does she know about his ogling, but that she quite enjoys it; that is all possible. But knowing Kathy, it's not that likely.

Unfortunately it just seems that her partner has a wandering eye, and I suppose I can't tell whether or not this brings his trustworthiness or fidelity into question.

I can't jump to any conclusions here, or talk about it with Kathy – I have learned the hard way that these things are better left up to a couple to work out, without the interference of a caring friend.

Ten years ago, I lost my best friend of 14 years due to a similar circumstance. Becky and I grew up together and spent our childhoods, teens and early twenties as close as sisters. We confided everything in each other: first period, first cigarette and first boyfriend. She was there for me when a friend of mine committed suicide; I was there for her when her ex-boyfriend was convicted of a violent crime. We were inseparable.

Naturally we talked about sex. We even discussed experimenting with each other when we were drunk and curious, and we laughed about it afterwards. Always supportive, we were a crutch for each other to lean on when love dealt us the pain of heartbreak. We cried a lot together, and we shared everything.

So when her boyfriend handed me his pager number one night, laid his hand on my knee and breathed into my ear that if I ever wanted a fuck, I should call him, my first instinct was to call Becky and tell her what he had said. She was totally besotted with him – I thought she would want to know that he had made a move on me. I was so wrong.

At first she was stunned and angry and was going to dump him, but that soon changed. When he lied and said I'd come onto him, she swallowed every word and dumped me instead. Our last ever conversation was him screaming down the phone that I was a 'lying cunt' and a 'fucking bitch' while she wept in the background and I was too shocked to speak.

I haven't seen her since, not for ten years. Happy end of friendship anniversary, Becky.

Of course I tried to rectify things with her. I spent months calling and writing letters, hoping that she would see some sense and know that it was him who was lying to her, not me.

She didn't want to hear, and shut me out of her life totally, staying in a relationship with him. The whole thing tore my heart apart; I felt the loss of her for many years.

I know that what happened says more about her being weak and an unloving, untrusting friend, than it does about me doing the 'right thing', but given the chance to go back in time, I wouldn't tell her what he'd done. Rather, I would warn *him* to watch his fucking back, that he'd better not hurt her *or else*, but I would let her figure out for herself what a prick he was. That way I wouldn't have lost my best friend.

Faced with this hindsight, I know that I cannot tell Kathy about her boyfriend's roving eye. It seems almost futile, and it's far too risky to be worth the bother. It makes me sad because I'd like to think that I am an open and dependable person who can tell the people I love what I think and feel, but given the danger of losing another friend, I think I'll just stick with wearing baggy tops and letting my shoulders slouch when I am in front of him. If my tits are less noticeable, he'll have less to look at and hopefully he'll rest his eyes elsewhere in the future.

Wednesday 22nd June

I'm still annoyed about Kathy's boyfriend's boob obsession. If there is one thing that pisses me off, it's when men in relationships give me the once over in front of their girlfriend or wife. I've got zero tolerance for it. Now I've learned to scowl as spitefully as I can at the perpetrators, especially if they make eye contact, or, God save them, smile at me.

It's not the looking that's a problem – like I said of Kathy, it'd be OK if she was in on the game – it's the looking without their partners knowing that I dislike. To me, this is an act of betrayal, and where trust, loyalty and honesty are the prerequisites to a good relationship, this duplicity lies very uneasily with me.

It's not the same as secretly having sex with another woman – obviously that's a far more serious misdemeanour; but to hide a fantasy is to keep a secret from one's partner and this retriction of truth sits very uncomfortably with me.

I was out shopping today and my local high street seemed to be full of partnered-up men looking at my body, smiling at me – furtively – as though they were indulging in their own private daydream, a momentary ego-stroke for them. Or wank fodder for later. It really annoyed me.

Maybe I get so riled because this is what it was like for me with my ex, Steven, and I was on the receiving end.

I always knew when he was looking at other women when we were out together. I remember being with him at a social event and he couldn't keep his eyes off a woman with big breasts. He was staring and staring at her chest and I could see the horniness in his eyes. I recognised it.

Seeing him turned on, turned me on. All I wanted was for him to look at me, wink and smile, and I knew that I would be part of his fantasy, that he was letting me in on his stiffening cock and his desire to fuck this other woman, that we could talk about it later when we had sex and both get off on it.

But he didn't look at me. He didn't notice the fire burning in my eyes. He didn't know that watching him, watching her, made me want him. He excluded me and continued eyeballing her, as if to get every detail of her embedded in his mind so that he could use it another time. Without me.

This exclusion made me feel rejected, unwanted and

undesirable and I became jealous – not a habitual emotion for me – of his attraction to her.

When we got home that night, Steven pressed me against the wall and I felt his dick against me. Although my body responded as it always does (fast breath, erect nipples, wet pussy), I felt troubled. When he lifted my top up and cupped my breast with his hand, I wondered if it was her he was imagining. When he slowly sucked on my nipple, I wondered if he was thinking of *her* breast in his mouth. When he eagerly entered me, I felt like it was her he wanted to fuck, not me.

Perhaps all these insecurities and reactions – rational or not – would not have happened if Steven had included me in his fantasy. If he had glanced over at me and smiled, or said 'She's got great tits, I'd love to suck on them and watch her suck on you; it would get me so hot', then maybe I would have responded totally differently. The fantasy would have then been about US getting off on it together, rather than just HIM. With Steven excluding me from this it made me feel like I couldn't really trust him. And as it turned out, I couldn't, given that he was fucking someone else, half his age, when he was seeing me.

Even though I'm cynical about all this, I still hope one day to meet a man who will be able to trust me and be open about his desires and kinks, and let me be open about mine. A man who'll know that being honest with me means he can be free to express himself and not be fearful that I would judge him or want to possess him. I want a man who will squeeze my hand on the street and whisper in my ear that the gorgeous woman walking towards us is making him get hard, knowing that it will make me want him even more.

Because a man who could do all this, is also the man who knows that he would have freer, more passionate, and wilder sex, than if he just smiled at women in the street when he was with me, and then secretly masturbated about them without me knowing. A man that knows all this is a rare breed indeed; he's a real man – and I haven't met one yet.

But I'm still looking.

Sunday 26th June

When I met up with Blog Boy last night, I thought the idea was to behave in a dignified manner and continue trying to maintain our 'let's just be friends' stance – after all, that's what he asked for. But after a few glasses of wine in the pub, when he leaned in to kiss me, it didn't cross my mind to fight the urge to kiss him right back. Nor did I want to; it all felt right.

After snogging drunkenly for ages, we left the pub arm in arm and got as far as the street corner before sinking into one another again, his tongue dancing in my mouth. Then he grabbed me by the waist, pulled me close and pushed his hands slowly down my skirt until they came to rest on my arse. He squeezed it tightly and I instantly got wet as I felt his hard dick through his jeans. I wanted to feel it in the flesh so badly …

We began to move against each other, the instinctive need to push and grind making us oblivious to our surroundings. As his hips matched mine, his hands moved upward and gently cupped my breasts through my top, and my fingers greedily explored under his shirt, discovering his firm nipples and his delicious chest hair. I was so turned on I wanted to take his cock out there and then, and suck it.

Then a car pulled up alongside, interrupting us rudely with a beep of its horn.

'Need a taxi?' the driver called out.

We did need to get somewhere more private, it was true, especially if I was going to fulfil my desire to get his cock in my mouth as soon as possible.

I looked at the man leaning out of the window of the estate car and eyed him suspiciously. 'How much to Clapham, then?'

'Twenty-five,' he replied.

I laughed. 'Do I look like a tourist, mate? No way. Pull the other one!'

'You won't get any other cabs out here at this time of night,' the cabbie said, dryly.

He was right. No other vehicles had passed us in the time we had been standing on the street – let alone cabs. But £25 for that journey made him a rip-off merchant.

I eased myself out of Blog Boy's seductive grip and turned around to face the driver, pointing at his empty windscreen. 'Mate, you don't even have a licence displayed; what you're doing here – picking us up on the street – is *illegal*.'

The cabbie looked embarrassed and said, somewhat defensively, 'No, no, I *am* legal, but I just … um, don't have the paperwork yet.' He looked at me hopefully and then added, 'OK, how about twenty, then?'

'Twenty? Are you serious? It's a tenner to Clapham, twelve *max*.'

The cabbie stared at me, shocked. 'Clapham is South London. This is West London. Twenty quid. You won't get it for any less than that.'

Blog Boy leaned over and whispered into my ear. 'He's right, you know. Maybe we should just get it.' He rubbed my bum tantalisingly and I wondered what his fingers would feel like if they slipped just a bit further round, between my legs.

I collected myself and got my business head back on.
'Nonsense,' I exclaimed, 'it's a rip off.' I turned back to the
driver. 'We'll do it for twelve, no more.'

'I can't do it for that,' he said. 'It's too far from here.'

'Fine,' I retorted. 'Goodnight then.' I flung my arms back
around Blog Boy and repositioned my lips against his. His
hands immediately found their way to my arse again and the
cab driver took the hint, speeding off into the distance.

'You know, we may not get another cab for hours,' Blog
Boy said, his fingers now slowly circling my breasts. 'And I
think we need to go somewhere *quickly*, don't you?' He
pushed his cock up against me, emphasising the point.

He was right. We had been standing on the street for the
better part of an hour. As much as I wanted to unzip him and
slide my hands around his penis and let him push his fingers
into me, I knew it would have to wait – at least for a little
while longer.

'OK,' I said, as my fingers stroked him gently through his
jeans. 'We'll get the next ride that comes.'

He nodded and twirled his fingers around my nipples,
kissing me hard. We resumed our heated entwinement.

Moments later, there was another beep of a car horn.

The taxi was back. 'OK, love,' the cabbie called, 'twelve
quid it is then. Get in.'

I grinned at Blog Boy and we stumbled into the car.

The cab sped off at the breakneck speed that is somehow
mandatory for unlicensed vehicles. There was cheesy eighties
music on the radio but Blog Boy and I hardly noticed. As
London zoomed past us in our race across town, we were
preoccupied with something more pressing – that is to say, his
fingers sliding gently into my crotch and my hand wrapping

around his cock. I wasn't thinking about the fact that we'd crossed *way* over the platonic line. I was wondering when he'd push his lovely long fingers right into me.

So much for just being friends then.

I couldn't wait and grabbed his hand to slide two of his fingers in to the hilt.

'Shall I put another in?' he whispered, kissing my neck.

I nodded, and he kindly obliged.

His cock pulsed in my hand and I lifted my fingers to my mouth to taste his pre-come. He saw me and smiled, and covering my fingers in my saliva, I replaced them back around his shaft, tracing the tip gently.

It was exquisite. With Blog Boy's hand deftly working his magic on me, I was in heaven. But there was a problem: I was very close to climaxing.

Normally, this would not be an issue: I rather enjoy having orgasms and, as you know by now, I am not the sort of woman to turn one down, given the choice. But we were in a cab and the driver was sitting two feet away. When I come it's pretty intense. I would:

Find it hard to be silent.

Shake a lot.

Possibly leave a wet patch.

So I tried to hold back because I didn't want the driver to overhear or watch it all in the rear-view mirror.

I didn't want the first orgasm I got to have with Blog Boy to be experienced within the confines of a taxi, either. I am a lady, after all. Or at least I'd like Blog Boy to think I am.

So I took my hand off his cock and tried to focus every last drop of concentration on controlling myself and delaying the building orgasm, clutching the seat and clenching all my muscles.

And, of course, I then came like a steam train, practically crushing Blog Boy's hand between my legs as I squeezed them together convulsively.

Clearly I have no control. But that's no surprise when I was at the mercy of his finger magic.

I was still in a post-orgasmic haze when we pulled up in Clapham. I was tidying myself up and hadn't had the chance to open my own purse, when Blog Boy pulled out a £20 note and handed it to the cabbie. He helped me out of the cab, telling the driver, 'Keep the change, mate.'

The cabbie grinned from ear to ear and then immediately sped off. I stared at Blog Boy, stunned. 'You gave him a twenty?'

He shrugged. 'Look, it was worth it – it was a long way to come. He deserved a tip.'

'But what about my haggling? I gave him the hard sell – he agreed to twelve.'

Blog Boy shrugged again. 'With what we got up to in there, I think a tip was needed, don't you?'

I wasn't so certain: surely my intense orgasm in the back of his car should have been the bonus, but I wasn't going to complain. Not now we were at the flat and were about to get naked and devour each other at last.

When we got upstairs though, I began to feel nervous. I felt totally unprepared to shag him: my legs and muff needed shaving and I was also mid-way through my period – wearing my most boring old pants. I was sure nothing was going to happen when I left the house that night, and now I was caught out.

We were about to see each other naked for the first time. Should I try my hardest to turn him on and hope he'd enjoy it? Or should I be passive and let him take the lead, so that he didn't feel undermined by my sexual confidence? Fuck, it was hard.

Blog Boy made it all easy for me. As he removed my skirt, he kissed me deeply, slipped a finger inside me and made me climax again. His delight as I convulsed from his touch answered all my anxieties – he liked me and got pleasure from being with me and that was all that mattered.

So I relaxed and we spent the rest of the night feasting on each other. It was fantastic; it felt natural and right, and when he kept whispering 'You're so beautiful,' over and over again, I believed him.

He had to go to work early this morning, so we left together. As we said goodbye on the train, I noticed a little awkwardness between us, a lack of conversation.

Then Blog Boy kissed me on the cheek and said 'Catch up with you soon,' which I thought was odd, given how close we had seemed last night. I don't know if I should read anything into it; maybe I'm just being neurotic – I don't know.

What I do know, is that if I didn't fancy the pants off him before, I certainly do now.

The Girl's Guide to Fuck-Buddies: *Definitions*

1 A fuck-buddy is someone with whom you are sexually involved, but with no romantic or emotional strings attached. They are NOT a friend that you fuck; although they might be someone you like and respect, the fuck-buddy relationship is purely sexual

2 Occasionally a productive one-night stand can lead into a series of regular one-night stands. These then develop into an occasional sexual relationship

3 Shagging someone with no expectations of commitment or co-dependency does not have to mean a one-off: it can also be pleasurable to have multiple sexual experiences with them over a period of time

4 There doesn't need to be any awkwardness, guilt or hurt; it should be a simple situation, with little or no complications. It is not a problem if you only want to see someone because you are horny; you don't need to get validation from them on an emotional or intellectual level. You can get that from your friends

5 With a fuck-buddy, there is no real intimacy beyond nudity and mutual horniness. You might have nothing more in common with the other person than sexual attraction. It's not like meeting up with a mate to watch a movie and talk about the plot afterwards over dinner. By definition a fuck-buddy connection happens on a physical level only

7

July

Saturday 2nd July

It's not something I talk about often, but here goes: my friend Fiona is a professional dominatrix. That is to say, men – and for her, it is always men – hire her to inflict pain and suffering on them. Not the most conventional of hobbies, I know, but for Fiona it's been part of her everyday life for many years.

Though I've known her since college, I have always turned a blind eye to what she did; I never really wanted to know how she earned her cash. I didn't like the sound of BDSM in the first place, but the idea that men paid her to hurt them was more disturbing. As far as I was concerned, out of sight was out of mind.

Over the years, Fiona has offered me the chance to sit in on a session several times so that I could understand what she did and get some insight into the fetish/bondage scene that she's involved in. I've politely declined her offer each time, and made do with just listening to her as she relished telling me sordid tales of her adventures instead.

Recently, maybe because I have been exploring so much lately, and because I've had the diary to read back over, I've become more curious. Who are these men and why do they crave abuse like that? And what is BDSM really like? So I plucked up my courage to ask if I could watch her at work, and she was really chuffed. It looks like she may have a session coming up soon. I am terrified.

Monday 4th July

If Blog Boy and I are to get any more involved – and I am sort of hoping that we might now since things have changed somewhat – I think he is going to have to understand that there will be three of us in the relationship.

I don't mean that I will have another boyfriend, or that he will have another girlfriend. Nor do I refer to our having a threesome with another woman/man, though obviously, I would not rule that out at some point, were he (fingers crossed) into that sort of thing.

No, what I mean is that besides my relationship with him, I would also be having a relationship with his cock.

It's not that I fetishise the cock over the man: I am learning that my attraction to a guy is more about his personality, intelligence and attitude than the way his penis looks in a pair of Calvin Klein kecks. No, it's the fact that as well as getting to know his innermost feelings and basking in his affection and love, I'll become more intimate with him by striking up a relationship with his cock.

I think there is something almost secretive, a private dialogue, in the process of becoming close to a man's penis. *He* might not be talking with me, but when my mouth is wrapped around him, his cock is certainly communicating.

When I was seeing Steven, I had a great conversation with his penis one morning:

I woke up early and Steven was still asleep, snoring for Great Britain. I was randy, and debated having a quick fiddle, then decided against it. I had a better idea.

Shifting down the bed and lifting up the duvet, I moved my face down to Steven's cock. It lay there, spent from the previous night's activity. 'Ugh, I'm tired,' it said.

I shifted my face onto his thigh. 'Yes, you must be exhausted,' I said quietly. I laid my hand across the shaft. 'Perhaps you should stretch out a little?'

His cock didn't move. 'I'm too sleepy.'

I moved closer so my breath grazed him. 'You're probably overtired. I can make you feel better." I pressed down gently and ran my thumb along the length of him.

He pulsed. 'I'm aching a little …'

Me: 'Perhaps I should kiss you, then?' I leant forwards and kissed the tip lightly, feeling him pulse some more against my mouth.

His cock: 'Yes, that's a little better.' He began to stretch out.

I felt his warmth against my lips. 'What about if I lick you? Would that soothe you a little?' I ran my tongue lightly along the shaft, dragging it softly across the skin.

His cock stiffened slightly. 'Yes, that's better; I'm beginning to feel more awake.'

I wet my lips and lowered my mouth to him, letting just the tip slide slowly in. 'How is that?'

His cock throbbed against my tongue. 'Mmm.'

I gave his cock another kiss. Suddenly Steven himself stirred. I lay absolutely still, not wanting to give the game away just yet, my mouth poised over his shaft. The moment passed and Steven continued breathing deeply, oblivious to my little *tête à tête*.

'Ssh,' I whispered to his cock, 'let's keep this to ourselves for now.' I hovered over him again, and slid the length of him into my mouth.

His cock got harder as it moved against my tongue. 'Yes, let's not tell him, it'll be our secret.'

I agreed, and pursed my lips and sucked him deeply, moving my mouth back and forth. I felt his cock swelling as I tickled him with my tongue again.

We continued in our clandestine liaison, until his cock was rigid and bouncing around in my mouth. At this point Steven lifted the duvet and looked down to find my lips wrapped around his penis. He looked at me as if to say 'What are you doing down there, darling?' and there I was grinning at him, as best I could with my mouth full.

Now he knew and I knew that I had been doing something without his knowledge, but his cock, you see, had been carrying on with me quite independently of Steven, who wasn't even conscious at the time.

If I had just woken Steven up that morning and suggested sex, he might have declined, because he was still knackered from the night before, but suggesting sex to his cock was another matter altogether. I exploited this to my advantage; I knew that a gentle, slow, teasing blow job could subtly persuade his dick to wake up, and then I was bound to get a good rogering from Steven. A win/win situation, in my opinion.

I know that indulging in sexual intimacy with Steven's penis without his consent, involved some manipulation and coercion on my part and I felt bad about this, but when an otherwise average morning began with a delicious blow job that left me, Steven and his cock very happy indeed, I really found it hard to feel guilty for long.

I'm a repeat offender, but no one else has complained about my despicable behaviour, so I can only assume that guys are content for me to have these private dalliances with their cocks. As long as they understand that my relationship with their penis will occur in parallel with, and simultaneously to, the one with them, life could be very easy, I think.

Although I find it's best not to speak out loud to a cock – that's just wrong.

Saturday 9th July

Last night Blog Boy and I were standing on Holloway Road kissing.

I love kissing. It's got to be one of the most underrated aspects of sex, and it's probably my favourite. A good kiss will get me going, no problem. A good kiss is like making love with your mouth. A good kiss takes me away to that place where the only things you can hear are our synchronised breaths as we part our lips, and the only thing felt is the pulsing between my legs as he presses against me.

Blog Boy is a great kisser. No, strike that: a fantastic kisser. His kisses send shivers down my spine, make my fingertips tingle and my pussy throb. His kisses make my whole body feel electric. His kisses make me forget who I am and what I am doing.

So that's why we were standing on Holloway Road, snogging like two drunken teenagers on a night out, oblivious to the people milling around us trying to get the last tube home. The warm summery air was making us both frisky: our hands explored each other greedily as our mouths moved in unison.

We stood there and kissed, and the world revolved around us. It was magical.

I was extremely aroused, and I knew from the way he was grinding his crotch against mine that he was too. Everything was intensified, so when he mumbled in my ear that he wanted to 'feel' me, I didn't question what he meant, and just went with the flow ... even when he squeezed his hand down the front of my jeans and twisted two fingers into me.

I don't know if it was because

a) he turned me on so incredibly much;
b) I am becoming such a sex fiend that doing something so risqué in public excited me;
c) he seems like such a well-brought-up boy, which makes what he did totally out of character, and that made it even more outrageous –

but within 60 seconds I was having a massive orgasm. As we stood on Holloway Road. With people walking all around us.

I did try to conceal what was going on, but it wasn't easy. When the shaking subsided, I suddenly came back down to earth and realised what had just happened. I was mortified and made him remove his hand and tried to compose myself.

I have never done anything like that before. If he had given me longer to think about it, I would not have let him do it, but because I like him so much and because of those glorious kisses, I didn't have time to think. Before I knew it he was fingering me in full view of London.

How he had the guts to do that, I have no idea. How I had the guts to let him do that, I have no idea. Maybe he thinks I'm the sort of girl who would be up for it and took his chances. It seems he lucked out; maybe I really am a sex fiend.

But no matter how dirty or sordid I might think I am, his audacity showed me he's far more willing to push the boundaries than I thought he would be. Even if he looks like butter wouldn't melt in his mouth.

Wednesday 13th July

I have a bone to pick with men.

It is not about the fact that some – OK, most – of them stare at my tits.

And it is definitely not about me wanting a shag and being pussy-teased by all the cute men I see, until I have to rush home to have a wank, although it is most inconvenient, especially at rush hour on the Northern Line.

No, what I must speak out about is a terrible, terrible crime. Men shaving their chests.

Stop it. Now. I mean it.

'Why did you shave?' I squealed at Blog Boy a few days ago, as I felt the stubbly regrowth under my fingertips.

'I thought that's what women wanted,' he replied, mystified as to why I was so disappointed.

Wrong, wrong, wrong. What women want is someone who'll let us unload our stress at the end of a hard day; who can give us sympathy and cuddles when we have PMT; and who will offer us a nice firm cock to do what we like with, on demand.

But depilating your pecs? A firm NO. That is not something women want. Ever. At least, not a woman like me.

Hair is what makes a man a man. Even just a sprinkle is sexy, though I personally prefer the full forest to the barren wood.

Recently I've encountered a couple of guys who shaved off, or aggressively trimmed their chest fuzz and this has begun to worry me: why do men think their hair is so unattractive to women?

I fail to understand why they do this. I love to feel it under my fingers – the bristliness and roughness contrasting beautifully with my own softness and smoothness. Let's face it, if I wanted to stroke a smooth chest I'd sleep with a woman – which although nice in its own way, is nowhere near as pleasant as being with a man.*

So please, I beg all hairy men: leave your chests alone. Stop worrying about women finding your hair a turn-off; a real woman will like you for who you are – fur or no fur. Allow yourself to grow bushy! Let your forest run free! Be the man you are – be hairy. Women like me will spend hours fondling your chest and love every minute of it.

If you blokes must shave or trim something, by all means chop off your pubic hair – it is, after all, not that pleasant getting hairs stuck in one's mouth mid-suck. The increase in sensation you'll feel will be huge – definitely a reason for trimming it.

Just think: you could get your balls sucked if they weren't lost in your pubes; you could feel a tongue dabbling around your shaft – its wetness soaking the skin where the hair would have been. You'd get regular blow jobs because it would just be *easier* for us girls to slide your smooth cock all the way into our mouths. Worth a try if you ask me. You'd certainly get no complaints from this girl were you to go hairless – my mouth would be far too occupied to actually speak.

With apologies to my lesbian sisters once more, but you are most definitely missing out here.

Monday 18th July

When I woke up this morning I was wet.

Not that this was anything unusual for me, since I always wake up horny, but this situation was different. Firstly, because it was only 5 a.m., and not a great time to be wide awake with the raging horn, and secondly because, not even three hours ago, I had been given three intense orgasms by Blog Boy, who was still lying next to me in my bed.

I looked over at him in the dawn half-light. He seemed to be sleeping, his gentle breathing rhythmically lifting his diaphragm up and down. I watched him for a moment and pondered my options.

I considered going back to sleep. I was, after all, very tired; that earlier session had drained me a little.

But I was still horny.

I couldn't understand it: it wasn't as if the sex we had hadn't pleasured me – it had – the powerful orgasms he had given me had more than satisfied me. I was deliciously content.

But I was still horny.

I lay there and felt annoyed with myself. Why can't I just be a normal woman? Why does my body have to plague me with this perpetual randiness? Why *am* I such a sex fiend?

I watched his sleeping face for a moment, and got a flash-back to his expression when he was in the throes of passion last night. I closed my eyes and remembered the joy of it, trying to relax my brain using that image, that beautiful post-coital moment of bliss.

But I was still horny.

I knew that sleep would evade me until I had let off a bit of steam, so I decided to have a quick fiddle.

I slid my hand between my legs and stroked. Jesus, I was wet. I couldn't recall the last time I was that wet; even my thighs were slick with my juices. I rubbed myself as I thought about all the sexy things we had just done, and I watched his face as I pressed my hand against myself, wondering what he might think if he knew I was playing with myself and thinking about him.

Suddenly he jumped out of bed. He was awake.

Startled, I turned and saw him standing by the end of my bed. For a moment, I thought he was putting on his clothes and was leaving.

My heart sank. Not because it was the first time in my life that a man had left in the morning, but because I was shocked and hurt that despite our friendship and despite how much I like him, he would scarper so early. Didn't he like the sex? Was I too demanding? Or was it because he knew I had been playing with myself, and was put off by my high sex drive?

It was because he had cramp. He rubbed his leg furiously then jumped straight back into bed and laid his arm across me. Clearly I am a neurotic twat.

We lay there for a moment and snuggled. I debated trying to get back to sleep.

But I was still horny.

With Blog Boy's arm on me, and knowing he was awake next to me, turning me on even more, I knew that there was no hope for it. I had to achieve some release.

I slipped my hand down between my legs again and told him I was playing with myself.

He lifted the covers to look for himself and moved nearer to me, resting his hand on my arse and draping a leg over mine. I couldn't bear it: I was so close. I needed *him*, my own hand wouldn't do the job. So I told him how wet I was.

He reached down and felt how slick I was and when he pushed his fingers right into me, I felt myself gush onto his hand.

As he deftly worked his fingers in and out, I felt him rub his thigh against my thigh – his cock pressing into my arse cheek – and the sensation was overwhelming. I knew I wouldn't last long. Within a couple of minutes I was having a mind-numbingly intense orgasm and as I felt him spurt against my bum, my body convulsed so fiercely that I felt like I was going blind.

We lay there afterwards, both grinning, the post-orgasmic thrill still pounding round our veins, and then, the nicest thing of all, he fell asleep. I had felt guilty about interrupting his sleep because he had to be up for work in a few hours. He started snoring softly after our explosive five o'clock quickie, and I was relieved and happy. At least something good – aside from the shag itself – can come out of being such a sex fiend, even if I had to sleep on our combined wet patches.

The only downside was that when he was leaving, Blog Boy told me awkwardly that we shouldn't have sex again, because we had to protect our friendship. He added that he was going to try to take a 'moral' stance and *behave* when he's with me. It seems like he doesn't want me to think that the fact that we fucked again means anything more to him than just that – a fuck.

After he'd gone, I lay in my bed and cried into the pillow. It still smelt of him.

Diary of a Sex Fiend

Tuesday 19th July

Spoke to Tim this evening. He has a knack of cheering me up and gave me a wonderfully supportive response when I sent him a picture of myself in shorts, vest and trainers, ready to go for a run.

'Abby, I gotta tell you, you look FIT!'

'Shut up, you.'

'Serious! I knew that you went training, but I didn't know you would look so good!'

'Honestly, be quiet, Tim. You're talking out your arse.'

'I'm telling you – that picture – you look really HOT!'

'Look, you saw me a few weeks ago; I haven't changed that much since then.'

'Yeah, but your thighs and arse were a bit bigger then. You're so trim now! Looking really good!'

'Well, thanks. But if you really think that from looking at that photo, you're mad.'

'You must have men queuing up outside your door.'

'Um, no. None at all right now …'

'What? Come on! There must be a few – looking like that, they should be begging to get at you.'

'No, sadly, they're not.'

'Not even one?'

'Can we change the subject, please?'

'Honestly, Abby, all the blokes you know must be fucking stupid or something. What the hell is their problem? A beauty like you shouldn't be single.'

'Thanks. Now can we change the subject, please? Got laid recently?'

'Fucking fools, the lot of 'em. I think you're fucking gorgeous, you know that, right?'

'Yes, and I love you for it, thank you, but if I ever get rich and famous I bet you'd sell our sordid sex tales to the highest tabloid bidder without hesitation, wouldn't you?'

'Of course. You know me.'

'Well, as long as you give me fifty per cent of whatever deal you cut, and make sure I come out looking good, I'm fine with it.'

'Don't worry, I won't tell them about you squirting all over my bed. Your wet secret is safe with me.'

'You mug. That wasn't me. That was the girlfriend you had after me.'

'Oh. Shit. Well, anyway, wanna meet for a beer next week?'

'As long as you don't stare at my arse, my dear, it'd be a pleasure.'

Shame Tim and I are so incompatible; he is otherwise a lovely guy and will make some woman very happy.

Especially given his devotion to eating pussy on a daily basis.

Friday 22nd July

Fiona called me this morning – said she had a client who wouldn't mind if I sat in during his session with her. So I set out to meet her at an address in the City this afternoon, feeling seriously uneasy about the whole thing.

The dungeon turned out to be nothing like I'd expected.

Instead of arriving at a Tower of London-type castle with a moat and a drawbridge, I found myself buzzing the intercom at the door of an average-looking block of flats. I breathed a small sigh of relief.

Fiona opened the door and led me into an inconspicuous

duplex: the top floor had a lounge, kitchen, two bedrooms and a study, but the basement was something else – room after room devoted to various forms of sexual play.

The dungeon where Fiona works was painted black, lined with mirrors, and two of its walls were covered, floor to ceiling, with every instrument of torture you could imagine: whips to paddles, ropes to chains. I had never seen so many of the things collected together and was a little dumbfounded by them. I didn't even know what half of them were for.

As I was looking at the tools of the trade, a non-descript chap in his mid-thirties entered the room. Fiona told me later that he worked in IT; he seemed totally 'normal' to me and was very polite.

In return for letting me sit in on his session, he had requested that I 'looked the part too' so the fantasy wasn't spoiled. I grudgingly agreed to wear the rubber dress and six-inch platform stilettos he handed to me as gifts. It felt wrong that they were presents; I'm not the sort of woman who accepts money or other handouts from men I don't know – it feels like prostitution to me.

The dress was very difficult to get on. Not only was it very tight, but the zipper ran from the chest down to the thighs, making it hard to do up once it was in place. Since it was obviously designed for a C cup bust, my DDs spilled out over the top when I finally wrestled the zip up. This, Fiona assured me, was a bonus in the world of S&M.

I then had to close the five buckles that ran across the zipper, from the top to the bottom of the dress. Not that there was much of a 'bottom' to the dress: it barely covered my arse – I was glad I'd thought to wear knickers.

So there I stood, barely able to breathe, in this skin-tight rubber dress, trying to balance in these outrageously high stilettos. I wobbled and took a look at myself in the mirror.

I was amazed at what I saw.

Until then, I had never understood why people fetishise rubber. As far as I was concerned, it was just weird. I mean, getting excited about a material? *Please.* Get a life. It's just a garment, for heaven's sake.

But now I finally understood: I looked HOT in rubber. The dress clung to every curve on my body. Its tightness was like a corset, holding everything in, and accentuating my figure. It displayed my breasts in all their glory, proudly cupping them as if they were the firmest, roundest bosoms in all the world. It gripped my arse, squeezing the cheeks together like two delicious hardboiled eggs vacuum-packed in black cling film. It smoothed my body into an hourglass, a shiny, sleek, utterly erotic form. I felt like a seductress and I loved it instantly.

Of course I didn't want to go next door into the dungeon, after that. I was turned on and I wanted to play instead, but Fiona came to get me and finally the session with the client began.

All last week Fiona had been reassuring me that I wouldn't have to participate in any way, but I still felt uncomfortable. All the pleasure I'd taken in the sight of myself poured into the rubber dress evaporated as I stepped out of the changing room.

I watched Fiona strap the guy onto a gurney. His hands and feet were bound with ropes and chains. OK, I thought, simple enough, nothing too heavy. I can cope with this.

When Fiona started slapping him around, I didn't think much of it either; I like to think I am an open-minded person.

But when Fiona tied some rope tightly in between and around the guy's testicles and then strapped them to a pulley, which hauled them above his body, I began to have second thoughts about the whole thing.

I could see he was in pain: his body was pinned down, his balls pulled up. They started to go purple. I felt sick as I saw him grimace and then moan.

Instead of releasing his balls, Fiona abused him verbally, humiliating him, calling him all kinds of names. When that didn't have the desired effect, she spat into his mouth. Yes, spat. Gobbed. Big ball of saliva. Into his mouth.

The guy just smiled at her and swallowed it. Fiona told him he was a good boy and then tapped her cigarette into his open mouth, as if it were an ashtray.

I thought about leaving at that point. Some pain I can understand, but to be abused like that – I found that very disturbing.

Somehow I hung in there – probably because my curiosity about human nature got the better of me.

After a while, Fiona undid the guy, leaving the rope tied around his balls, and he moved to another contraption, a type of half-table. He was duly strapped face down to that with some leather cuffs and Fiona proceeded to use some of the 'toys' I had seen lined up against the wall earlier.

I lost count of the different instruments she used. Various whips, paddles, canes, crops and wooden rulers. There was a lot of blood, and his backside was criss-crossed with welts.

It looked excruciating but at the back of my mind I was trying to convince myself, Each to their own. Don't judge others just because you wouldn't do it.

Fiona got out a latex strap-on dildo and then proceeded to fuck the guy up his arse with it.

Although I found the idea of this disturbing, I realised that watching a man being penetrated was exciting for me too.

It showed me that:

a) I like to watch sex
b) I like penetration of any sort, either watching, doing or
   being done to
c) I want to fuck a man up the arse myself

I found myself getting turned on again by the thought of
doing this to a guy – although I saw myself being less aggres-
sive, far more gentle.

But when she pulled the strap-on out of his arse and
forced the guy to lick his own arse juice off the condom, I
thought about getting out of there. I thought I'd reached my
limit then; I couldn't overcome my revulsion.

Luckily the session was almost at an end, but before it
could finish, there was the small matter of his orgasm to
contend with. Throughout the session, his cock had been
totally flaccid, and I had wondered if the whole S&M dominatrix thing was just a mental fantasy, especially since Fiona
swore that she never performed any 'sexual' acts on her clients.

I was wrong. Fiona told the client she wanted him to
orgasm, and he got hard immediately. She then instructed him
to climax on cue, and so he grabbed his cock and wanked
himself off in front of us, finally climaxing as she commanded.
He spunked a wad all over her latex-clad hand, which she then
shoved into his mouth. If I hadn't been so repelled, I might
have been impressed by the way she made him ejaculate on
command, but I was pretty sick to my stomach by then.

Here was an average bloke, dependent on paying someone
to get his rocks off. Someone who would never love him, who
would always abuse him. I couldn't get my head round it. I

have no interest in being abused, or abusing another to such an extreme.

But seeing Fiona in action and, surprisingly, feeling myself respond to a few of the activities has me intrigued about experimenting with a little light S&M for myself.

Tuesday 26th July

I now have a fetish to go with my obsessions – the sex one and the lingerie one. Not rubber; although, yes, obviously there is that now, but not only that. You see, I have discovered I have a thing for men in suits.

That's right, suits: buttoned-up shirts, stylish ties, smart trousers with matching fitted jackets. Anything that makes a man look like he's going to work – serious work. I'm not sure when I began to find this attractive, but it's got more and more appealing over the last few months.

I do find my new weakness odd, because a suit is so intrinsically conservative. It represents everything I dislike so much about the Establishment: the suit is the uniform of all capitalist moneymen and bullshit politicians.

But then it's not so much what the suit represents as what lies beneath it – the male body. Maybe it's the contrast between the two: the cut, rigidity and conformity of the clothing juxtaposed with the hidden texture of a man's body hair, his muscular curves and the hardness of his cock.

Or perhaps it's just that it seems so tantalising to see a guy fully suited and booted, with his erection pressing up against the fly of his smart, pressed trousers: his carnal desire contrasting with his otherwise restrained appearance.

It makes me think of a mild form of bondage: the shirt

buttons tight across their chests, the tie choking them, the trousers squeezing their genitals – just like the rope I saw Fiona take to that IT specialist. To me suits are the male equivalent of a short rubber dress and platform heels: everything's packed in tight and it is hard to move, but *damn* is it a good look!

When I see a man dressed in a suit, it makes me want to rip his jacket off, pull him roughly towards me by the tie with one hand, while whipping down his zipper and freeing his cock with the other. To have him – and his suit – at my beck and call, a reversal of the power that this uniform seems to epitomise, is tantalising to me.

Then there's that air of authority in a suit. I don't mean in the traditional 'this man is obviously brainy and important' way. Rather, in the dominating 'throw me down on the bed, tie me up and spank me' kind of way; something that I know I now want to experience.

It seems to me that being smartly dressed not only allows a man to be elegant and appear important, but it also gives him a mask to hide behind. Like the sharply dressed, James Spader in the film *Secretary*, a man in a suit appears to be polite and decent, but given half a chance he'll pull his cock out of his tailored trousers, bend his girlfriend over the desk, and fuck her hard from behind. Elegant and rampant together – yes, please.

And that's why I can't stop watching the men in suits when they pass me in the street. Are they a normal, everyday guy who likes football and beer, or, are they the intense, thrusting, craven man who wants to tear off his suit and give his wife a good seeing-to?

Sadly, most of the men I meet don't wear suits, and those I meet who do are more the type of bloke who has to take each piece of clothing off one at a time and fold it neatly before entering into any nookie. A passion-killer if ever there was one.

So for now it's just a fantasy: the lover who will turn up at my house wearing an immaculate new suit, unzip himself and tell me to 'suck it', before bending me over in front of him and fucking me ruthlessly whilst slapping my arse. It's a damn good fantasy, though. Maybe I shouldn't be too hasty in dismissing it.

Where was it that all those City boys hang out again?

Friday 29th July

It's been almost two weeks since Blog Boy and I last slept together and I still haven't heard from him. I know I shouldn't be feeling this way. I know it's pathetic, but I'm hurt by this lack of contact.

I guess it's silly of me to think that having sex with him meant anything – I know a one-night stand when I see one, after all, but I thought something was developing between us. Am I totally wrong?

Blog Boy said he wanted to be friends and not fuck-buddies, then he slept with me – three times – and now I don't hear from him at all. Not even a text to say hello – as a mate.

I finally emailed him today to wish him well on his holiday – I think he leaves tomorrow. He replied, somewhat blasé, and wished me a good summer.

So much for our friendship then – let alone anything else.

It seems like he now has no interest in me at all; so why do I care so much?

Sunday 31st July

I wasn't expecting a threesome last night. In fact I wasn't even expecting a *twosome*. I *was* expecting to get well and truly slaughtered on cocktails with Fiona. I really, *really* wasn't expecting to end up in bed with a total stranger and a professional dominatrix, but that was where I found myself, a few hours into the evening.

At some point on our cocktail crawl last night, it had got to the point where both Fiona and I were wobbling unsteadily, giggling madly and talking absolute nonsense. We discussed my sex life and my frustration at the lack of adventure. There I was, prepared to experiment and eager to try out new things, and yet I still hadn't experienced any S&M. I was gutted – surely *everyone* has experimented with some light bondage and spanking by this point in their life?

So I moaned, and Fiona cut me short by asking me what I thought of a guy at the end of the bar. He was well built and fairly good-looking, tall and blond too, so I gave Fiona a drunken, 'yeah, I would'. She grinned at me, and, being a generous sort of girl, asked me whether I wanted her to pull him for me.

This didn't make sense; I mean, if I wanted to shag him, I could have asked him myself. I wasn't sure why she was offering to oversee the whole process. She looked at me with a sly look on her face, and said that I was going to try something new tonight, and that she was going to invite him to join us in it.

Now Fiona is my friend – we aren't lovers. Nor am I interested in being sexually involved with her. Not that she is unattractive or unsexy to me. On the contrary, with her auburn hair and blue eyes she's quite the opposite, but I have a little rule that I like to stick to, and that is **I do not fuck my friends**.

Sleeping with Harry all those years ago I learned the hard way that, at best, shagging your mates always results in some kind of confusion and plenty of complications. At worst, someone gets hurt or feels too uncomfortable to continue the friendship. In the past this has resulted in me having one less friend in my life – a sad sacrifice to make for a night (or nights) of passion – and I don't plan on doing this again in a hurry.

Real life is *not* like a movie, where two best friends end up making out. Real life is embarrassment and nervousness and insecurity, and waking up the next morning and realising your friendship may never be the same again. Real life is losing your best friend of 20 years because you got drunk together and fooled around. Real life is where you are nervous being alone together even though you've spent your childhood sharing a bed with this person. Real life is where you're not sure whether your friend is looking at you because they want to rip your clothes off or because they think that skirt doesn't suit you. Real life is about making sure boundaries don't get crossed and sex and friendship are kept separate.

So it was with some hesitation that I responded to Fiona's suggestion that we have a threesome together. She swore blind that it wasn't that she had some kind of unrequited love for me, nor was it because she was dying to get into my pants. Rather, she was offering to let me experience some S&M under her protection – so that I might finally know what it was like and tick it off my list. She argued that if we had sex, it didn't need to *mean* anything because she didn't fancy me. She was just offering to help me out, nice friend that she is.

Boozed and a bit horny, I said, 'Yeah, whatever,' and left Fiona to work her magic with the guy at the end of the bar. Not many people say 'no' to Fiona. She is the most assertive woman I know; her personality is so magnetic that even if you found her point of view disagreeable, you'd soon find yourself coming round to her side, because she leaves you no other option.

That was exactly what happened to this man: he never stood a chance. A short time later I was in his bedroom with Fiona, watching him strip off his clothes.

He stood there naked, looking at Fiona and me, somewhat wary. I wasn't quite sure what to do either. Was there some kind of etiquette I should know about? Who goes first, who touches whom where, who is the 'toucher' and who is the 'touchee'? This could be a minefield, but Fiona had a game plan and she suddenly became Mistress F – and the bloke and I were going to follow all her orders, *or else*.

Fiona told me to get undressed and lie on the bed. I took off all my clothes except my bra and pants and moved towards the bed, but I didn't do it quickly enough and warranted a quick sharp slap on my arse from Fiona's hand. Ouch! It hurt, but the sting felt good somehow – it throbbed almost pleasantly.

I felt my arse cheeks smarting and lay on my front, quickly. Obviously this wasn't to Fiona's satisfaction either, she whacked my arse again, but this time the pain seemed more direct, more focussed. I was aware of something more than her hand moving through the air and heard something crack. I turned my head to see that she now had his belt in her hands and it was still swinging after she'd used it to lash my poor bottom. The pain changed from an intensely sharp sting to a warm soothing pulse. I rubbed and it felt sensitive to my hand, the skin tingling as I caressed it. *Nice.*

Fiona crawled up onto the bed with me and whispered in my ear, 'Are you OK, do you want to play like this?' I looked at her, my friend, and knew that I could trust her unconditionally. I replied 'Yes' and that was the last Fiona/Abby conversation we had with each other until the whole episode was over.

Fiona turned me over and grasped both of my hands above my head. In a matter of seconds she had them expertly tied together with the belt and strapped to the bed. My wrists hurt and I grimaced slightly. This earned me a quick slap on the face, then she stuffed the guy's t-shirt in my mouth as a gag and pulled apart my legs.

Now she removed my pants and bra and was hovering over me, grinning. She pulled off her own top and bra and sat on my stomach so I could barely breathe.

'Are you a good girl?' she asked me.

I nodded. She slapped my face.

'I said, are you a good little girl?'

I nodded enthusiastically, scared of what Fiona might do next.

'Good girls don't make a noise when I do this,' she said, and then grabbed my nipples so hard I thought I would scream. But I just bit down on my gag and tried to endure, thinking to myself that it would all be worth it.

Fiona moved down my body and knelt between my legs.

'Spread them,' she said, and I opened my legs as far as they would go.

'Mmm, nice pussy,' she remarked, 'good girl, you keep it nice and trimmed,' and she pressed her fingers against my labia.

I wondered if she was going to do something painful to me and I flinched as she stuck her fingers inside me, aware that my excitement was increasing with her touch.

'Good, you're nice and wet,' she said and removed her fingers. 'Come here, Slave,' she called across to the man.

All this time he had just been watching, busily stroking his cock, probably thinking he was going to stand on the sidelines and see some girl-on-girl action. He hadn't reckoned on Fiona, though.

'I said come here, Slave. Now.' Fiona stood up and walked over to him. 'Bend over you little slut!' she shouted, and he did as he was asked.

Fiona whacked him so hard even *I* could feel his pain: my spanks were nothing in comparison to what he was getting. She carried on spanking him for a while and when she felt he was getting too vocal, she slid a hand between his thighs, gripped his testicles *hard*, and whispered in his ear:

'You little piece of shit, you don't make a fucking sound unless I tell you to, you don't move unless I tell you to. You do everything I tell you to. Do you understand?'

He nodded.

'And you call me Mistress, got that?'

He nodded again.

'Right, now you're going to go over there, lie between Abby's legs and eat her pussy until I tell you to stop. Do you understand?'

He nodded once more.

'And don't even think about letting this get soft for one minute' – she gripped his cock tightly – 'We'll be using this shortly. I want it hard all the time. Got that?'

He had no choice but to nod – she had him by the balls.

When Fiona let him go, he got onto the bed with me and ate my pussy hungrily.

With his head eagerly lapping between my legs, Fiona dealt out occasional slaps sharply onto his arse. Then she moved over to me and removed the gag from my mouth, replacing it with her breasts, which she pushed forcefully into my mouth. It was strangely unerotic – not that I dislike sucking on some nice breasts – far from it, especially not large ones like hers – but it was Fiona, my friend, and that was too weird. I think it was for her too; she removed them and resumed walloping the guy's arse instead.

After a while, Fiona grabbed him and pulled him up over me, so that his cock was parallel with my mouth. She bent over to me and grabbed my face in both her hands.

'You're gonna suck his cock now, like a good girl. Do as I say and I won't punish you.'

I nodded meekly. He looked very excited at the prospect of some oral action and began to move in towards me.

Fiona almost ripped his arm out of its socket and dragged him backwards.

'I didn't give you permission to move, did I? No. You'll start when I say. And don't even *think* about coming yet, I don't want to see *any* spunk on your cock, do you understand?'

He nodded nervously once more.

Fiona grabbed hold of his cock and pulled him by it until the tip was pressing into my cheek. She gently wiped it against my face and across my lips, and then slowly slid it into my mouth, before standing back and alternating between thwacking him on his arse and slapping me on my face.

I was choking a little; it was only natural, sucking hard on a cock that had been crammed into my mouth when I was lying on my back, but it wasn't unpleasant. I felt trapped and yet free, scared and yet safe, simultaneously freaked out by what I was doing and yet amazed and delighted at the same time.

I was tied up, unable to move, gagging on a mouthful of cock, and yet I felt *unbelievably* horny. It was the weirdest feeling to be *so* passive, and yet still be able to pleasure someone else. I realised that I liked it.

So when Fiona pulled his cock out of my mouth, rolled a condom onto it and shoved it into my pussy, 'making' the stranger fuck me, I laid back and let myself become part of the surroundings, part of her, part of him. I didn't think about getting off, I wasn't bothered when an orgasm was going to happen: I was focussed on the calmness of my mind, the physical freedom that I felt and the pulses of energy that were surging through my body. I don't know whether I had an orgasm or not; my whole body felt like one big climax and the sheer power of what was taking place in that room was enough for me.

This morning, when it was all over, Fiona and I left the stranger to sleep and went to have a good old English fry-up in a greasy spoon. We laughed about what had happened and I thanked her. Since watching her work in the dungeon, I had wanted to experience BDSM; last night I finally discovered what it was like.

I've learned that I really enjoyed being submissive, that it isn't something to be ashamed of and that a little light roleplay never hurt anyone.

Well, my arse still hurts, maybe, but it was worth it.

The Girl's Guide to Fuck-Buddies: Rules and Regulations

1 Mutual respect is a prerequisite. If you are going to be fucking the living daylights out of someone, you should have the decency to keep to any arrangement you make and be on time for the event, or, if you have to cancel, do so well in advance so they can make other arrangements

2 If you are only planning on having a brief shag before going on elsewhere, it's only decent to let the other person know that you are slotting them into a 'window'. This will help avoid disappointment since they may have been hoping for a long night of passion. Remember a quickie can always be rearranged if necessary

3 There is no need to spend time discussing the other person's day/work/boyfriend/girlfriend/politics, etc. You are not there to debate the weather; you want sex with them. Tell them that; cut to the chase, make the most of the time you have and enjoy

4 Likewise, if you are going to call, text or email your fuck-buddy during the week, don't make idle chit-chat. Instead, talk dirty to them; tell them you can't wait to fuck them, arrange the next meeting and then get off the phone/internet as soon as possible

5 Don't apologise for wanting sex; be polite, flirtatious and firm. Make it clear from the outset that you do not desire any emotional attachment and check that the other person feels the same. Mutual consent = good sex.

8

August

Wednesday 3rd August

I am a fool. I contacted my ex, Steven, today.

Tim had told me about a party happening this weekend – another swingers' thing. I am really eager to go, but have no one to go with. It can't be Tim, because neither of us wants to risk our friendship by having sex with each other, or find ourselves as frustrated as we were at the spa.

After considering all my options: Tony – has girlfriend; Tom – not in London and back with girlfriend; Ben – in Manchester; the young guy – too immature; Franklin – too fragile; the journalist – too emotionally confused; Blog Boy – out of the country and possibly disinterested in me; I realised I had no one left.

So I decided to email Steven and invite him. Not clever of me, I know. But a sexy swingers' night might be just what I need right now, so I dropped my standards momentarily.

I wrote him a brief note, making it clear what I wanted:

'I can't think of a better way to end a fun evening than to be lying handcuffed on the bed and have you easing your cock into my mouth, before you fuck me hard. I am wet now just thinking about it. We had some great sex together: it would be nice to spend a night fucking each other again.'

I explained why I was inviting him:

'I would like to go with someone who I know I'll have fun with, who I enjoy having sex with, and whom I can trust; and not because I want anything more than that from you. Accompanying me to this event would involve having a laugh and enjoying having no-strings-attached sex with me – and maybe others too – all night long. Nothing more. There is no catch.'

And I meant what I said. I am past the point where he can hurt me emotionally, or where I would feel uncomfortable being intimate with him. I would be ready for whatever happened, whether he said yes or no.

But I didn't expect this response:

'I know it's not very smart of me to turn you down, but I spend my weekends with Petra these days and don't want to jeopardise what I have there.'

Petra is the 19-year-old that he was fucking whilst he was seeing me. Hearing that he was now spending his weekends with her made me think one thing: prick. That's it. Just prick.

You see, the worst of our break-up was the knowledge that he was sleeping with someone who was more than ten years younger than me. I went through the predictable self-loathing and doubt that women who are cheated on go through:

★ Is she prettier than me?
★ Is her body sexier than mine?
★ Is her pussy tighter than mine?
★ Is she better in bed?
★ And, what does she have that I don't?

Dumb, I know, but I couldn't stop myself demanding to know why he wanted to be with her – surely I was enough for him?

Then it dawned on me, it was far less to do with me, and much more about him. Here was a man who was almost 40 and incapable of having a meaningful relationship with a woman his own age. A man so shallow and so lacking in self-esteem that he had to have sex with a girl more than half his age to feel better about himself.

I'm not denying that it might be a buzz for any older man to get a teenage girl into bed or that most men would leap at the chance if it fell into their lap, but knowing Steven and how badly he actually felt about himself, I know it was more about his feelings of worthlessness than about his sexual prowess and his ability to pull a young woman.

And so, in the last few days we were seeing each other, I got over my self-loathing. I realised I was beautiful, I was sexy, I was good in bed – and I had a tight pussy (15 years of doing Kegel exercises certainly pay off). As a woman closer to his age, I knew that the qualities I could offer him – intellectual stimulation, emotional understanding and loving acceptance – were far beyond anything a teenager could provide. She would lack the worldly experience to be a real partner to him.

Rather than feeling angry with Steven for cheating and being so emotionally immature, I felt sorry for him instead. I knew he had problems, I was aware of the issues, and I tried to accept his baggage and work at a relationship, but it didn't pan out.

So even though I sent Steven that invite, I was half expecting him to turn me down because he couldn't cope with seeing me again – my emotional maturity may have been too threatening for him.

I was even ready to hear that he was seeing someone else; I hoped that he was pulling his life together, too – being healthier, meeting a good woman and falling in love again. That would have made me happy for him. I do want the best for him.

But hearing that he is now spending his weekends with Petra made me feel angry, because he never even gave up his weekends for me. The fact that he added, 'I have never been very good at lying so I cannot look her in the eye and come and meet you for the night,' was like a slap in the face. He lied constantly to me about shagging her, seeing us both on the same day, sometimes.

So, I don't even feel sorry for him any more. I think he is pathetic and disgusting and totally shallow. I am glad I am not with him. I am doubly glad that I haven't had sex with him again.

It was suddenly all in perspective: I have absolutely no desire to be with someone like him. He is no longer attractive to me, emotionally, mentally, or physically.

And just like that, he was out of my mind. I couldn't think of him while masturbating again; it'd make me feel quite ill. I don't find him appealing at all. I don't have feelings for him now, and I don't care about him as a mate any more. I just don't give a shit.

This is a shame because I like to stay friends with my exes – some of my good male mates are people I have been intimate with and I love them to bits, but I have no desire to ever see or speak with Steven again. I couldn't be friends with a man like him, and why should the fact that we used to fuck change that?

It was like a mental spring clean; instead of getting rid of those old books and CDs that I was never going to read or listen to, I got rid of Steven. I no longer want to recall the first time I did anal with him, or the time he gave me more than 20 orgasms in one night. Thinking about those occasions doesn't turn me on any more. I've moved on. I want to forget that part of my life.

And I have. I feel free. And happy. I have learned from this experience and grown as a person.

But it would still be great if I could just erase those memories like they did in that film, *Eternal Sunshine of the Spotless Mind*, and flog the data that's wiped from my brain. It'd be a much neater way to close this particular chapter in my life. Plus, given the wealth and variety of sordid material in there, I bet I'd make a fortune.

Saturday 6th August

Even though I'm gutted about not finding someone to accompany me to the swingers' party this evening, I am actually beginning to long for some good, clean, simple fun once more – normal, boring, one-on-one shagging – just like I had when I was 18 and going out with Chris.

Back then he would stay over most weekends, and we'd barely make it out of my bedroom, venturing out only occasionally for food, drink and a quick shower. The rest of the time we spent sleeping, talking and, of course, shagging. Though there wasn't much privacy because I was still living at my parents' place, we still managed to get through boxes of condoms in our voracious lovemaking.

During one brief break, I remember staggering downstairs with him one evening. My parents had gone out and we had the house to ourselves. Dressed only in towelling robes, we began to snack to fuel our appetites: peanut butter on toast for him, Marmite sandwich for me. Being English we had to have a nice cuppa too, and I brewed up the kettle to make a big pot of tea.

As it boiled, Chris sat down behind me and called me over to him. I turned around, and he was grinning at me. I smiled back at him and followed the direction of his gaze. It led, of course, to his crotch. I looked closer, and through the towelling, I could see a bulge. He looked back up at me, smiling even more and, with one small motion, undid his robe and grasped his cock in his hand.

I stood there for a moment, pondering his erection, and then decided to walk towards him, letting my own robe fall open.

I slid myself on top of his thighs so that his cock was pressed up against me, and pushed my breasts into his face, like I knew he loved it. Sucking furiously on my nipples, he grabbed my arse hard, and ground himself against me until he could feel I was slippery enough to take him. Lifting me by my hips, he swivelled and adjusted my position and then pulled me down onto his cock roughly. He moved in me deeply; I felt him pulse and knew that both of us were near.

As we were about to climax, I heard 'Oh, sorry, Abby! We didn't know you were … um … in here. Er … ' and I turned my head to see both my parents backing out of the kitchen, blushing furiously.

Chris and I were stunned. Our bodies said it all: moments before at the point of orgasm; now numbness, softness and all that pent-up ardour went straight out the window. There's nothing like the anti-aphrodisiac of one's parents walking in to kill the moment.

With shame on our heads, we shuffled back to my bedroom, and kept ourselves hidden from view for many hours. I was too embarrassed to face my parents properly for days.

This incident was never discussed or spoken about, but I knew that they knew exactly what we were up to, and in my opinion, that's a little bit too much information for them to have embedded in their brains.

Still, it didn't put Chris and I off: we were back shagging again some hours later, albeit with less gusto and noise. He had a great appetite, that boy.

Thursday 11th August

Hello, my name is Abby, and I am a sex fiend.

1) I have admitted I am powerless about sex – my life has become unmanageable.
   Frenetically masturbating at every given opportunity is rather inconvenient.
2) I have come to believe that a power greater than myself could restore me to sanity.
   Who would have known that Duracell Extra Strength could last so long?
3) I have made a decision to turn my will and my life over to the care of God as I understand him.
   I'll gladly give up my will; handcuffs and ankle restraints might help.
4) I have made a searching and fearless moral inventory of myself.
   The use of a compact mirror often comes in handy.

5) I have admitted to God, to myself and to another human being the exact nature of my wrongs.

Screaming out his name just as I am about to climax is the best admission of all.

6) I am entirely ready to have God remove all these defects of character.

Returning over-used broken vibrators to their maker is my speciality.

7) I shall humbly ask Him to remove my shortcomings.

Although I am all for the quickie, I do prefer the longer, more drawn-out climax.

8) I will make a list of all persons I have harmed, and be willing to make amends to them all.

For all those I gave rushed blow jobs to, I thoroughly apologise; it was only because I was going crazy not having your cock inside me that made me hurry so.

9) I will make direct amends to such people wherever possible, except when to do so would injure them or others.

For all those I gave rushed blow jobs to, and who are now partnered-up with someone else, I thoroughly apologise; you'll now just have to imagine my lips around your cock, sucking you for an hour.

10) I will continue to take personal inventory and when I am wrong, promptly admit it.

I promise to throw out all my other sex toys and only keep the most effective one.

11) I will seek through prayer and meditation to improve my conscious contact with God, as I understand Him, praying only for knowledge of His will for me and the power to carry that out.

If asked nicely, I will gladly worship a cock; clasping my hands together and bowing my head when requested. Crucifixes are optional.

12) Having had a spiritual awakening as the result of these steps, I will try to carry this message to other sex fiends, and to practise these principles in all my affairs.

★ *I will try to spend less time looking at pornography, and more time on foreplay.*

★ *I will try not to judge the fuckability of all men I meet; I can be just friends with men.*

★ *I will try* to spend my free time doing artistic and creative things, rather than always ending up with my hands between my legs.*

Wednesday 17th August

There are times when single women like me may have difficult conversations with our mothers. They might begin with, say, 'I'm pregnant,' 'I'm a lesbian,' or even 'I'm thinking of becoming a nun and living in isolation, far away from the family, for the rest of my years.'

Yes, my mum and dad walked in on me and Chris having sex in the kitchen, but as I said, we preferred to brush the incident under the carpet and never mention it again. So explaining the difference between vanilla and BDSM to my mother was not something I ever expected to do.

The conversation started off innocently enough. We were talking about the forthcoming wedding of Billy, a bloke I work with. Moving on from the normal issues – who's going,

---

*But twice a day is still necessary, or I'll go insane.

what I should wear, what present I should buy – my mother and I ended up disagreeing about the groom.

I thought he was young, dumb and full of come, and may eventually cheat on his bride. His serial long-term monogamy has limited his sexual experiences, thus leaving him in possible need of self-discovery via casual shagging with other women.

My mother, however, disputed that, stating that perhaps he is satisfied with his wife-to-be, and that not every man needs to shag around and rack up notches on their bedposts.

I pointed out that I've noticed his wandering eye at work – he's always flirting with the actresses on set – and suggested that at some point, he might follow things through with one of them. Again, my mother argued that just because he might look at other women roguishly it didn't mean that he would actually have an affair.

I was quickly losing this argument. Damn my mother and her open-minded progressive outlook! I raised the stakes. I ventured the opinion that I imagined their sex life to be very 'vanilla' and that at some point he may wonder what else was out there for him to try.

'What's vanilla?' my mum asked.

I stared at her and registered what I had just said.

'Is that when white people will only have sex with other white people?' she looked confused. 'Isn't that rather racist?'

Bless my mother.

'Um, no.' I replied. 'Vanilla is the opposite of BDSM.'

There was a pause.

'What's BDSM?'

I dropped my head in my hands and couldn't believe that I was going to have to describe it to her. Of all the things to talk about with your mother, kinky control play was not at the top of my list.

I tried to explain it succinctly: 'BDSM stands for Bondage Domination Sado-Masochism.'

She looked blank. 'What? Say it again.'

I groaned quietly. 'BDSM is Bondage Domination Sado-Masochism. Ways of exploring sex that are considered transgressive.'

'Ah,'' she said, 'so vanilla must mean boring, then.'

'No no, not at all. Vanilla just doesn't include, well, props, or role-playing and stuff like that, but it's still great. You know, missionary and things like that.'

I realised I was trying to pitch vanilla sex to my mother, and now I know exactly what that expression about teaching your grandma to suck eggs means. In this case, replace granny with mother, and eggs with cock, get an image in your head of your parents together, and you suddenly don't want to be having this conversation any more.

I tried to change the subject swiftly, steering it towards the location of the ceremony. My mother looked at me studiously and then said 'Have you ever done BDSM then?'

If the ground had opened up and swallowed me, to be honest it wouldn't have been enough. I did not for one moment want to explain to my mother about my recent foray into BDSM and how I'd enjoyed being handcuffed, spanked and fucked hard from behind. Nor did I wish to tell her about the time I watched a guy being whipped and then sitting on his face till I climaxed repeatedly. I especially didn't want to share with her my desire to dominate a man with a strap-on dildo. No, I didn't wish her to either know, or picture any of this, in any way.

So I was economical with the truth. I told her that I knew

of BDSM and was broad-minded about it, but essentially my tastes were vanilla.

Thankfully she then dropped the subject and we returned to the wedding, but as we talked, I'm sure I noticed her glancing at me oddly. It may be my imagination, but I'm beginning to worry that she suspects I have become obsessed by sex, and if she asks me if I am, I'm not sure that I could deny it.

Monday 22nd August

My love life is in a dire state of affairs (so to speak) just now. It's been more than a month since I've spoken with Blog Boy, who could be on the other side of the planet for all I know. It seems clear from the lack of contact that he's not interested, even in friendship, so it's futile trying to push things any further with him, much as I'd like to.

I haven't got naked since the BDSM threesome with Fiona and the man from the bar a month ago, and guess what? I'm gagging for it again.

It would be easier for me if I was at least dating, but the usual route – meeting people through work – is no longer fruitful because the freelance work I do has all but dried up.

I've also ruled out being introduced to a nice guy through my friends, who are mostly coupled-up themselves. Either all their acquaintances are married already, or – more horrifically – their taste has plummeted since they themselves got hitched.

Men that my friends, when single, would have not wasted four minutes of breath on are now 'lovely, friendly, and funny' men, even though they have the social skills of a Neanderthal and the intellect of a twelve-year-old.

I can hardly bear to mention the times I have been fixed up with men, whom I was told were 'interesting, warm and open-minded', only to discover that that actually meant that they owned 200 lesbian porn DVDs, had no female friends at all and were unable to look me in the eye when they spoke to me.

I would love to erase, for her sake, the recommendation that Kathy gave me about a man whom she described as 'really nice, caring and sweet', when what she really meant was 'he is unable to connect on any emotional level whatsoever and has huge hang-ups about sex'.

Let's not even delve into those 'I've heard he's good in bed' cases to which Fiona gave her stamp of authority: the supposed tiger she nominated for the shag of the century turned out to be the only wet pussy in my bed that night.

So, work and friends are out. Where else can I meet a man?

Well, there's the fallback option of pubs and bars I suppose, but though there might be the occasional choice bit of man totty on display, the amount of quality men in my local pubs is pretty non-existent.

I have considered – and tested – other means of meeting men too. I have attempted to approach the handsome man in my local supermarket; I have smiled at the geeky-looking guy in the gallery; I have given my phone number to a friendly man who sold me a t-shirt on a market stall – none of these paid off (gay, married, had girlfriend).

So I have decided to be proactive and try something else. I'm debating joining a proper internet dating service after my chat room experience a few months ago. There may be freaks, weirdos and psychos signed up too, but I bet they don't outnumber the ones I've met 'in real life'.

With a good dating site I would get to vet their appearance, learn about their interests and hobbies, and perhaps even find out their political viewpoints too. Though I have fucked a couple of Tories in the past, I don't plan on indulging any more.

Not that offensive politics make someone bad in bed – far from it – if anything, the arguments can make a good shag even more passionate. But the thing is I'm beginning to think that sexual ability is less important than a man's political beliefs: after all, you can always work on your bedroom technique, but your deeply-held political philosophy? I don't think so.

So, political matters aside, how do I work out how to write a profile for the dating site that will attract the right kind of man?

Stating that I think I have become a sex fiend might get me lots of dates, but would any of the men I met be interested in finding out a bit more about me, other than what I was like in bed? Likewise, writing 'multi-orgasmic' in the 'skills' box may get me a lot of offers to test out my abilities, but perhaps wouldn't enable me to show that I also have a brain and have occasionally been known to make people laugh too.

It seems that in order to write an eye-catching profile, one has to be a skilled marketeer, presenting oneself as a product with a distinct customer base. I'm crap at this sort of stuff: where do I fit in? What's my target audience? Apart from seemingly having a high sex drive, what on earth do I have to offer?

Somehow, I don't think including the facts that I am 'neurotic, insecure and perpetually self-analytical, due to being intermittently emotionally fragile' would be very good selling points.

Nor stating that I am 'highly opinionated, judgmental, and a smart-arse know-it-all' would win me any offers of a second date, I'm sure.

So what the hell do I write?

I have been wondering about using 'Sarcastic socialist seductress seeks similar soulmate' as a tag-line; it needs work, obviously, but it gets the point across, and surely I will impress many fine men with my clever and ingenious use of alliteration.

The discussions about possibly wanting kids at some point and dabbling in threesomes together can wait, I think.

At least until the third round of drinks, anyway.

Saturday 27th August

'She's just like you,' Tim said, as he took a big gulp of his beer.

'How so?'

'She'll never say "no" to a shag.'

'You have a tactful way of insulting me, you know.'

'Sorry. What I meant, was that like you she's always up for sex.'

'Ah, I see,' I winked at him. 'Always horny, then?'

'Always wet, you mean.'

I laughed, 'Definitely like me then.'

We paid for another pint and moaned about the portion-size of the food, wondering if we had ordered enough for our beer-induced drunken hunger.

'So, will you be needing Viagra, then?' I asked sarcastically.

He laughed. 'Not yet, though I did wonder if I'd ever shag again the other night.'

'She rode you hard? A woman after my own heart, obviously.'

'Well, she'd already made me come three times, and to be honest I was a bit knackered at that point. When she asked if we could have one last go before we went to sleep, I wanted to say no.'

'Ha ha ha. Sounds familiar. Did you tell her to have a wank instead?'

'Hell, no. A beautiful woman in bed with me, dripping wet; are you kidding me? It didn't take me much to get hard again, I can tell you.'

'Good for you. Glad to see you appreciate what is obviously a quality woman. Was it worth it?'

'Definitely. She came as soon as I slid my cock into her. I love that. Took me fucking ages to come, but it was a good pay-off at the end, even though I was fucking shattered.'

'Nice. You lucky bastard; it sounds lovely. That's what I need: a man who'll go the extra mile because they enjoy taking advantage of my sex drive.'

'What about Blog Boy? What's happening with him? Your little public display on Holloway Road sounded hot.'

'It was … but I'm not planning on being on display like that again in a hurry. I'm a good girl, don't you know.'

'Yeah, of course, I forgot. But you are far more daring than me. The closest I got to doing something in the public eye, was eating her pussy as she was standing at the kitchen sink with the curtains open.'

'Doing your washing-up, no doubt, you lazy bastard.'

'Well, she was very wet, but not from having her hands in the water.'

'She sounds like your type of woman, alright. So are you still looking to play then – got any couples lined up?'

Tim looked down. 'Um, no, I've stopped that for the moment. But if she wanted to dabble, I wouldn't say no; though I think we need to let things settle before we involve others.'

'Oh my. Here's a woman with a great sex drive, you enjoy her company, find her funny and sweet and don't want to fuck anyone else right now. Should I be buying a hat and fixing a speech?'

Tim laughed. 'Not just yet, but watch this space. I really like her.'

'I'm so happy for you. You deserve it. That really is great news.'

'What about you, then – what *exactly* happened with Blog Boy?'

I sighed. 'I don't know. He said he didn't want to get involved, he didn't call after we last had sex and now he's away on holiday, so I guess that's it. I should have known better really. Anyhow, I'm trying to stay positive. Something will happen at the right time, just maybe not with him. Until then, whatever happens, happens. I have an open mind.'

'I was going to say "and an open pussy too", but figured you might hit me if I did.'

'Cheeky bastard!'

We both roared and then Tim's expression became more serious.

'I want you to meet her, at some point; I hope you'll like her.'

I smiled at him, 'I'm sure I will. But don't be getting any ideas about the three of us in your bed.'

'I won't, don't worry. You're safe with me.'

'It's not you I'm worried about: if she's hot, I'll be wanting to bed her too!'

He smiled again, 'Abby, whatever man you do eventually end up with, he is going to be one lucky – and very happy – bloke. Just remember that.'

'Cheers, my dear. I'll drink to that.'

The Girl's Guide
Are You a Sex Fiend?

1 Do you regularly have your hand between your legs when you watch TV, talk on the phone, sit on the computer, etc?

2 Do you need to climax to relieve tension, stress and anger as well as for sexual pleasure?

3 Do you always wake up horny and need to have a good frig to start the day off properly?

4 Do you like to masturbate to send you off to sleep?

5 Do you find that you need to play during the day as well, and desperately sneak off into the toilets at work for a quickie?

6 Do you look at porn to get you off?

7 Do you get aroused by looking at somebody on the street?

8 Do you get aroused by pretty much anything?

9 Can you climax in three minutes flat?

10 Do you think about sex all the time?

If you answer 'yes' to five or more questions, then you are a sex fiend like me and there is no hope for you.

9

September

Thursday 1st September

'Would you please stop looking at my tits!' I pleaded with Kathy's friend as he attempted to dance in front of me.

'I'm not,' he retorted, his eyes still glued to my bosoms.

'Yes, you are – look!' I pointed at the direction of his gaze, which was focussed on my nipple line.

He quickly averted his eyes. 'See, I'm not looking,' he said defensively, his eyes immediately reverting back to breast level.

I stood there and raised a single eyebrow at him. Pointing at my breasts, I asked him, 'Do I look blind? You haven't been able to keep your eyes off them since you began talking to me.' I shook my head in disbelief.

'But they're just … you know … there', he pleaded, gesturing towards them, adding, 'I can't help it!'

I looked down at my non-low-cut, non-revealing formal blouse and watched him try to give me direct eye contact and fail. All he could do was glance from my tits to somewhere near my eye line and then back again. He looked up at me and shrugged hopelessly. Clearly this man needed help.

He had spent the last half an hour trying to chat me up. Trying, being the operative word, since his technique was severely lacking. Unable to remove his eyes from my chest area, he had barely been able to maintain any form of conversation and had had to ask me to repeat everything I said. I knew that if he used this technique on another woman, he was risking being ignored at best, or, and this is more likely, getting a big slap. So I decided to help him.

'Look, um, what did you say your name was again?' I asked.

'Gregory,' he replied, asking that I emphasise the latter consonants in his name. Interesting, I thought, this attention to his own personal details; and ironic that he could then overlook the necessary basic social skills when it came to women.

'OK, Gregory,' I said, rolling the other consonants off my tongue as if I were practising my favourite dabbling technique on the underside of a cock, 'this is how it is: you are not to look at my tits from now on. Got that?'

He grimaced and looked at my tits.

'You must be able to give me eye contact – try it,' I pleaded.

Gregory stared at my face with all his concentration. Three seconds later he was staring at my boobs again.

'Honestly,' I groaned, 'you're just not trying, you're pathetic ...'

He shrugged, and looked back at my tits once more.

'For fuck's sake, Gregory, do you really think that is the way to win women over? Is that your tried and tested pulling technique?'

He mumbled something incoherent and tried to focus on my face. I watched his eyes slowly lower themselves to my bosoms again and I knew that I was fighting a losing battle.

'OK, enough. We're going to have to try a different tactic. I want you to look at my tits.'

He looked up at me. 'Really? No, I couldn't possibly ...'

'Seriously, I want you to stare at them, really get an eyeful. Go on, look at 'em.' I glanced down at my chest, hoping his eyes would follow.

He stared at me, speechless.

'Come on, Gregory, take a good look, do it. I know you want to,' I said, in my most seductive, persuasive voice.

'Really? Are you sure?' he asked shyly, his face going a little red.

'Yes. Go on, look. Have a really good look.'

He still seemed unsure whether I was being serious or not and his eyes flitted between my face and my breasts awkwardly.

'Do it, Gregory. Look. I want you to get a really good look, because that's all you're gonna get. For the next thirty seconds, you are going to look at my tits, and after that, you will not look at them again. Understand?'

He nodded slowly.

'Right. Now look at them.' I lowered my hands to my breasts, cupped them through my blouse and gently squeezed them together.

Unsurprisingly, he lowered his eyes to my hands and stared at my chest, his gaze fixed.

'That's good,' I said, reassuringly. 'Look at them. Have a really good stare. Picture them in your mind, memorise every curve, each outline.' I removed my hands and looked at my watch. 'Fifteen seconds left.'

He stared – a man possessed – his expression one of awe mixed with excitement. I watched his mouth turn into a wide smile.

'Five seconds.'

He bit his lip and his eyes wandered across my chest.

'Time's up.'

He looked up at me.

'Right. You've had your look, yes?'

He nodded.

'And you can recall them clearly in your mind, every detail?'

He grinned.

'OK, good. Now, pay attention: whenever a woman is speaking, or you are talking to her, you must look her in the eyes, just as you're doing with me now. Do you understand?'

He nodded again, his eyes levelling with mine.

'There are two exceptions to this rule. Number one is that you can look at her tits, but – and I cannot state how important this is – *never* when in conversation. *Only* when she is looking away. Got that?'

He nodded enthusiastically.

'You mustn't even *slightly* glance at her tits whilst either of you are talking; don't think you can get away with a small sneaky peek – you can't. Women always know when guys are staring at their breasts and they'll rate you as a class A arsehole if you do it. Still with me?'

'I think so,' he said. 'So I can look, but only when her head is turned, right?'

'Yes. Like this,' I turned to look at the dance floor. 'You can look at my tits now, but as soon as I turn my head back, you need to give me eye contact again.' I turned round to face him once more.

He was staring at my eyes.

'You're learning; excellent. You've got to practise this. You'll get better, trust me.'

He looked at me excitedly. 'Fantastic. So I can look at her tits, but as long as she doesn't catch me looking, it's fine?'

'Something like that, yeah.'

'So what's the other exception to the rule, then?' he asked, somewhat gleefully.

'Ah, well, that's simple. If you're sitting in a darkened corner, her tongue is down your throat and her hand is on your cock, stroking it, then you can take it as a given that you can not only look at her tits, but you can cop a good feel as well,' I answered.

He laughed, 'You are an amazing woman. How do you know all this stuff?'

For a moment I considered telling him about my experiences so far this year and all the different men I've shagged. Then I decided not to: it would have been pointless, plus he wasn't someone I wanted to add to my fuck list.

'Let's just say, I have a few male friends and I do my best to ensure they get laid, because many of them are hopeless with women.' I quickly added, 'And if you make sure you don't stare at another woman's tits like you have at mine tonight, I'm sure you'll do just fine.'

'You should be charging for this,' he said, 'men would pay good money for advice on how to pick up women.'

I laughed at the irony of the situation – I'm broke and there's not much film work to be had – and I wondered whether he might be right.

Sunday 4th September

A girl can have too much of a good thing. Not sex, obviously. I can never have too much of that and I'm having a bit of a dry spell at the moment. No, I'm talking about condoms. I have far too many of them; it's as if my bedroom has been invaded by a pharmacy – they're everywhere.

It's not like:

a) I have any need for so many condoms given that I haven't had sex for over a month now;

b) I am a prostitute and can get condoms as a tax break;

c) I am planning any orgies where I'll need such a huge variety of prophylactics.

No. Most of these condoms will stay tucked up in my flat, never to see the light of day, or fulfil their short-lived latex destiny of being inserted deep into a very wet me.

The variety I have managed to collect astounds me. Alongside the Durex staples of 'Extra Safe' and 'Fetherlite' (thin) that I have purchased, I also have their more interesting 'Sensation' (studded) and 'Pleasuremax' (studded and ribbed) varieties.

Then there are boxes of Trojans 'Ultra Pleasure'(thin), 'Her Pleasure' (ribbed) and 'Shared Pleasure' (warming lubricant) that have been given to me free by some safe-sex marketing people. (Query: why don't they make 'His Pleasure' Trojans?)

Added to which are the freebie NHS condoms I have been handed during gynae' check-ups: Condomi 'Nature', and Pasante 'Naturelle', 'Trim', 'Regular', 'Large' and 'Extra Strong'.

And as for flavours, how about blueberry, strawberry, orange, lemon, mint, chocolate and vanilla?

Every type, every size, every flavour: too many. Too many condoms altogether.

Now I like to think I am a progressive woman because I believe in safe sex being a 50/50 split between both partners. I always have condoms at home, and like to give a guy the choice of type, seeing as he'll be the one wearing it.

But this can be difficult: I want a guy to know I am a liberated, modern woman who comes prepared for any eventuality, but when I pull open the bedside drawer to reveal 100-odd foil-wrapped condoms ready for use, he might think me a little strange at best, or a sex maniac at worst.

This could make for awkward dialogue in the heat of the moment:

Me: 'So, do you like ribbed? Or maybe silicone-lubricated? Or perhaps flavoured?'

Him: 'Anything is fine, just hurry up!'

Me: 'You're not XL are you? It's just that I've run out of those …'

Even with all this variety, when the 'condom moment' arrives I have learned that it's far less about 'What type is it?' and much more about 'Just roll it on quickly, I want to fuck you now.'

Not that I am against enjoying condoms as part of foreplay – not since I discovered that I can put them on using my mouth, at any rate – but breaking off to ask a guy what variety he'd prefer, kind of kills the mood, I think.

Ninety-nine per cent of the shags I've had, have proved that one size really does fit all, so I guess it doesn't matter what you use, as long as you use something.

I'm having a bit of a clear-out in my flat just now, so this is on my mind. What should I do with all these excess condoms? I don't think I need the huge selection? I can't bear to throw them away unused, though; that kind of waste offends me. I'm not getting enough action to use them all up just now. I wonder if my local charity shop would accept a donation?

Anyway, when I next have some rampant sex chez moi – and please *God* let it be soon – I think I might just ask the guy if he has brought any of his own instead. That way I can get to find out what he likes and make sure I am well stocked up with that brand for next time.

Though, obviously, one box will do just fine. A 12-pack, naturally.

Wednesday 7th September

I have met someone. Well, when I say met, I mean talked to. And when I say talked to, I mean we've exchanged loads of emails over the last few days. The profile I put up on the internet dating site seems to have finally paid off: a lovely guy has contacted me. Maybe it's time that I forgot about Blog Boy.

Like me, Jamie reads the *Guardian* and is left wing. He has a great sense of humour too – perfect. Thinking he might be too good to be true, I asked for photos. I was fully prepared to get some mug shots of a fat, ugly, middle-aged guy, but the shots he sent showed a good-looking guy in his early thirties. Another tick to the list.

When he suggested meeting today, I jumped at the chance. Things look hopeful, I thought, as I made my way to Café Nero in Soho.

Jamie turned out not only to be devilishly handsome and with wonderful green eyes, but he also had a dynamic personality. He was captivating company – even better in real life than in his emails. He was totally blasé about sex too, and talked about it frequently and openly. My kind of man indeed.

His jokes had me in fits of laughter, and as I noticed the lines around his eyes crinkling with warmth, I found myself fancying the pants off him. My body responded warmly to him as we sat spinning out our lattes, and aside from wanting to fuck him senseless, I couldn't help wondering if he wasn't Potential Boyfriend Material as well. It felt good to be meeting someone new and exciting and I didn't want to rush it, but enjoy it at my leisure.

So I only flirted with him lightly and gently teased him about the way he glanced at my cleavage, and when he put his hand on my waist to kiss me goodbye, I leaned in and squeezed his hip gently – little touches that said a lot. We agreed to meet up for drinks in a couple of weeks. By the time we parted in Soho I was wearing damp pants and a huge grin and I hope he had a decent hard-on too.

When I got home, there was an email from him waiting for me, saying how great it had been to meet. I replied straight away, saying how much I'd enjoyed meeting him too.

I know I shouldn't be crossing my fingers about this, or raising my hopes when it's early days, but it is looking good so far, I reckon.

Especially since my pants are still wet from thinking about him.

Friday 9th September

Dear Man on the Street,

We need to talk. There are some things you should know and I hope I can shed some light on them for you.

When I walk along my road, it does not, as you may presume, give me pleasure to be shouted at just because you have spotted my breasts and approve of them.

Contrary to what you may think, it does not make me

happy to have your eyeballs transfixed onto my tits. Staring, ogling, drooling – none of these make me appreciate the male gender. In fact the opposite is true: when faced with a man unable to tear his eyes away from my chest area, I am more inclined to think 'arsehole' than 'knight in shining armour'.

I know this may come as a shock to you. I assume you think that when you shout at me, 'Nice tits!' that I just *love* the attention, but you are wrong. Very wrong.

Let me explain:

★ It is not a compliment
★ It is not a turn-on
★ I do not go home and rub myself into oblivion, thinking how sexy your words made me feel
★ Your behaviour does not tempt me to drop my pants in front of you and say, 'Oh please, I love it when you say that, fuck me now!'

The only time anyone has a right to remark on my breasts is when someone like Blog Boy is in bed with me, and tells me how much he likes them, and then asks me to rub them against his cock. Then and *only* then do I like them being talked about, stared at and fondled. Any other time is just not on – *especially* if you are a stranger looking at me in the street.

You might think that I have no right to say these things, considering my own preoccupation with sex, and the delight I take in looking at men's crotches, but I beg to differ. When I look, I observe *subtly*, and hopefully never get caught doing it. I wouldn't dream of staring blatantly at a man's package or saying something out loud to him. Intimidating or offending him would be derogatory, and I would hate to make him feel objectified.

You seem to think that the reverse does not apply to you, and that your behaviour is acceptable. It seems that as a man you're free to say what you like about women's bodies when you like, and more often than not it's offensive. It makes me think that maybe hardly any men have actually seen real live breasts close up, let alone felt them. Why else would you behave this way? Surely you know better than to be so rude? How do you expect me to respond?

So, I hope that this will clear up any bewilderment you may have experienced when you heard 'Arsehole', 'Wanker', and 'Tosser' shouted back at you today. It wasn't personal, love, promise.

Yours truly,

Abby

Monday 12th September

'You have the feet of an angel.'

I turned round to find a thirty-something man in a suit grinning at me.

'Excuse me?'

'I said, your feet, they're angelic – so beautiful.'

I looked down at my feet. Granted, the turquoise nail polish I had on was cute, and the sparkly flip-flops quite sweet, but my size eight-and-a-half flat feet, angelic? I think not.

I looked back up to find him smiling contentedly at me. 'You see, lovely; they really are gorgeous.'

'I think you're mistaken,' I replied, adding 'but thank you anyway for the compliment.'

He shook his head. 'No, no, no, it is you who is mistaken,

you have perfect feet – I saw them from over there,' he gestured towards the tube station I'd just emerged from, 'and I just had to tell you how lovely they were.' He grinned widely at me.

I looked back at him, trying to mask my suspicion with an ironic arch of a single eyebrow, but quite probably looking like I was grimacing instead.

'Don't think I am weird,' he said, cottoning on to the exact thought running through my mind, 'it's just that, well, you are a very foxy lady, so I wanted to talk to you anyway, but when I saw your feet, I just had to say something, because they are the most gorgeous ones I have ever seen.'

I laughed. 'Well, thanks; I'm not quite sure I agree, but cheers.' I shifted my feet uncomfortably, aware that his gaze kept dropping to my toes, and for the first time in my life, finding it somehow more disconcerting that a man was looking at my feet, rather than my breasts.

'I know this may sound a bit forward, but, um, could I massage them for you sometime?' he asked, his eyes lighting up a little.

Oh great. A foot fetishist: just my luck. If it's not a breast-fixated man, or an emotionally unstable guy, it's a bloke who wants to worship my feet. Fabulous. I must have a sign on my forehead that says 'Only approach this girl if you are odd, an arsehole, or just plain weird. Normal guys need not apply'.

'No thanks,' I replied, 'though it's very kind of you to offer ...'

'Is it because you have a boyfriend?' he asked, pursuing the matter.

'Yes,' I lied, thinking that he would take the hint, 'he wouldn't really approve.'

'Oh, but there don't need to be any strings attached, I just want to stroke them,' he reasoned, thinking that this would win me over instead of causing me to bolt away down the road as fast as possible

'Thank you, really, I'm just not interested,' I said, adding, 'but five gold stars for your approach; the most original I've ever encountered.'

He grinned. 'Well, your boyfriend is a lucky man. You really are quite beautiful you know, and I hope he spends all night caressing your lovely feet.'

'He does,' I lied, thinking that if that was on my list of requirements for a partner, I would be destined to be single for the rest of my life. 'He's a lovely man; I'm on my way to see him now.'

He shook my hand and wished me well, and I walked off in my flip-flops, trying to appear both elegant and on-the-way-to-see-a-boyfriend, and so tripped over my own feet and almost fell right over.

It didn't seem to matter. He was still staring contentedly at my feet, a look of awe and delight on his face.

Thursday 15th September

Karl emailed me today, almost two years after we last saw each other. It's hard to keep in touch now that he lives in America. We're not close friends but Karl and I have, over the years, got together many times to have sex. Friendly fuck-buddies, if you will. We are very familiar with each other's bodies and he was the first man that I gave a blow job to and enjoyed it myself.

Up until my mid-twenties, I felt as though every blow job

I gave had been forced on me. Fellatio, as far as I was concerned, involved some form of coercion. Every time I put a man's penis in my mouth, it reminded me of some nasty occasions when I had my head pushed down onto a guy's cock so that it almost suffocated me.

Every time I did it, I felt disgusted. How could something so revolting turn a guy on?

Even when my boyfriend Danny, whom I cared for deeply, stuck his cock in my mouth, I hated it. I dreaded the moment when he would ask me to suck him.

That is, until I met Karl.

Karl is a hell of an attractive man. He has fabulous brown eyes and the sexiest laughter lines around them. He is intelligent: we used to sit up all night arguing about politics, him pro-capitalism, me pro-socialism.

We used to have bitter rows. We'd fight and fuck, and boy was the fucking good. Very passionate. Very heated. Very political.

Me *(riding his cock, digging my nails into his chest)*: 'You surely don't believe that the pursuit of financial wealth is the answer to America's problems? As if by making all poor people rich, you'll get rid of class oppression or racism?'

Him *(grabbing my hips, pulling me deeper onto his cock)*: 'You just want to tax everyone and stop people having the money they've worked for and that they deserve. Why should poor people get handouts? They should just work harder. That way they'll have the same chance as everyone else to be happy.'

Me *(pumping him hard)*: 'Oh, just shut up and fuck me.'

And so he did.

Karl wasn't just verbal, he had a few other favourite uses for his mouth too. He ADORED cunnilingus. To this day I have never met a pussy worshipper like him. He would beg me to let him put his head between my thighs and eat me all night.

Back then I was not such a fan. I mean, I would never say no to being licked and I did enjoy it, but given a choice between some labia-tonguing and a hot, hard cock thrusting in and out of me, it was always penetration that got me going every time.

Anyway, making Karl beg and plead was all part of the game, and he'd get stuck in, head down, like he hadn't had a meal all day. Gold star for enthusiasm.

I would watch him, and I began to notice that his cock would be flaccid when he started licking me, but that within a few minutes he would be grinding himself against the bed, rock hard. When he came up for air, his cock would be stuck out like a fucking flagpole.

I would grab him immediately, and try to fuck him, but he would always ask for just a little bit longer 'down there'. OK, whatever, I thought, as I lay back and got licked some more.

Knowing that he got a boner from eating me out turned me on, and it made me think: why did he enjoy it? I never enjoyed sucking cock. What was it that he liked about licking me? I gave it a lot of thought. Was it because I tasted nice? Or was it because he knew *I* was getting turned on as he did it?

Whatever it was, he got off on getting me off, and I realised that I had been being selfish. For some time I had just laid back with him working away busily and I had never given so much as a thought to sucking his cock. Karl had never even asked me to suck him, let alone pushed me down there against my will, like other guys had. Maybe because of this I wanted to explore him too and give him back some pleasure in kind.

Karl has the most beautiful penis. He keeps the area so

clean that I can still recall how sweet his cock and balls smell and taste as I write this.

It was only when I sucked him off that I understood how few blokes seem to wash properly, or frequently, and how if they had paid as much attention to their genitalia as Karl did, and kept it all so neat and trim, then perhaps the blow jobs might have been more enjoyable for me.

With Karl lying on my bed and his cock and balls all shaved and clean, I decided to lick him. He tasted good. So I licked some more, this time lightly flicking over the head. Karl moaned a little.

OK, going well so far. I licked from the tip to the base. Karl shifted his hips slightly, so his balls were under my tongue. So I licked them. Karl's breathing got faster. I opened my mouth and drew his balls into it. Karl gave an approving sound, so I sucked them a little. He moved again so that his balls were above my nose. I sensed Karl wanted me to go a bit further, and so far, things were going OK.

I wasn't on the verge of puking; Karl's breathing was heavy and his cock was rock hard. All good then. I licked the underside of his testicles, making him shiver. Then I moved down and nuzzled my nose against them. He groaned. I nibbled the base of his cock and licked the space between his balls and his arse and he bucked his hips, gyrating so hard that he was spasming against me.

So I decided to alternate between sucking, licking and nibbling the head of his cock, sliding as much of it into my mouth as possible, gripping it with my hands, lashing it with my tongue and swirling my tongue around the underside of his cock, balls and perineum.

And I was rewarded in more ways than one.

Firstly, Karl was going absolutely crazy: thrusting his hips in the air, groaning loudly.

Secondly, I was soaking wet.

I didn't know if it was turning Karl on that had got me horny, or if it was just having something so delicious happening in my mouth that aroused me, but I was desperate to fuck him senseless.

Karl read my mind. He grabbed me and pulled me up over him, easing me onto his cock. We rode each other for a few minutes, then climaxed together. Lovely.

So when Karl contacted me today to tell me he will finally be in town again soon, I got rather excited. I'm in dire need of another good hard shag right now, but I'm also looking forward to a good row. Not about politics though; this time it'll be over who gets to suck the other first.

I can't wait.

Wednesday 21st September

I am a hypocrite. A charlatan. A fraud.

I have made a mockery of everything I wrote about not getting caught looking at someone's cleavage. I got caught.

It was all going so well. Charlie and I had been working together for the last few days on a small project and we were getting quite friendly. Not *overtly* flirtatious, but there was still a hint of sex in the air – a suggestion; and while we're not indulging it right now, there's a distinct possibility that we'll explore it more fully in the near future.

Essentially, I was hoping that a shag would be on the cards. When he walked in this morning wearing a v-necked t-shirt I couldn't stop myself looking at his cleavage. I'm not talking about man-breasts – extra flesh in the male mammary department is not something that appeals to me. I am talking about 'man-cleavage', the hair on the chest that shows above his collar or through a gap in his clothes.

Just as the sight of a woman's breasts pressed together makes me want to plunge my hands in, so a hint of chest hair over a t-shirt neck, or revealed by an undone button, looks like an open invitation to run my fingers through the fuzzy mass.

Charlie had gorgeous cleavage, his chest hair rising right up out of his t-shirt, and tickling the underside of his neck, pushing against his collar like a soft furry lining.

It was driving me crazy. All I could do was wonder what he would look like with no clothes on, just a glimpse of it was a delightful pointer to what lay beneath. Every time he leaned forward the cotton hung loosely down and I got a view of his chest, and that pelt of glorious hair. It was mesmerising. I couldn't help but stare.

At some point he bent over towards me, and I found myself with a clear view of his nipples. I was filled with an incredible urge to reach out and touch them, and caress them through the fur. Just seeing this previously hidden gorgeousness made me want him; didn't he see what he was doing to me?

Clearly he did, because when I looked up at his face, Charlie was staring at me: he had caught me ogling his cleavage. Nothing would change the fact that he knew I had been staring at his chest; not even a quick flick of the eyes to his face, the ceiling, the floor. He knew, and I knew that he knew.

I felt myself going red, and all I could do was grin at him stupidly. To my relief, he grinned back. Somehow, we then ended up having a serious discussion and thankfully the moment seemed to pass with no further embarrassment.

Later on I caught him glancing at my boobs, which, ironically, was actually a relief to me, since I knew I'd been a bit out of order gazing so intently at him. I deserved some of my own medicine. Especially since I'm sure he caught me actually drooling.

Monday 26th September

As luck would have it, I was reminded of Karl again today – but not in a way I would have liked.

My dad had decided to download some software that sorts and displays every picture on your computer into nice neat little folders; very helpful.

What's not helpful is when the software finds an erotic photo of me which Karl took years ago and which has since lain dormant and long forgotten in the depths of the hard drive. And then the software blows it up in all its full-colour 17-inch glory on the screen before my father's eyes.

He called me into the room. 'Abby, I think you should see this.' He motioned towards the screen.

There I was, half naked, dressed only in stockings and a thong, facing the wall. My arse proudly displayed for all to see, my long brown hair flowing down my back – a dead give-away. It was pretty clear who the semi-clad model in the picture was.

I had a sudden flashback to the night in question. Karl ripping my clothes off, seeing my lingerie and begging me to let him capture the moment on camera. Me hiding my face out of shot, him snapping until the film ran out. Karl then removing my thong and eating my pussy for half an hour and finally fucking me hard on the kitchen floor. God, it was a good shag.

Back in the present day, however, my dad was looking at a photo of my bare arse. Oh shit. Fuck. I couldn't deny it. That butt was mine. 'Erm. Oops. God, I didn't even know that was on there. Er … ha ha?'

He carried on facing the screen. 'What's that doing on my computer? Who took it?'

I remembered Karl emailing it to me years ago when I didn't have a computer – I can't believe I downloaded it onto my dad's machine. As Dad waited for a response I racked my brain and tried to come up with the most valid and feasible answer I could think of.

Nothing sprang to mind. 'A mate took it. I forgot he sent it to me. Thank God it's just my arse, eh?' I tried to laugh it off.

Then my mother walked into the room. Oh great. Both my parents are looking at a picture of me wearing stockings and a thong, sticking my butt out sexily. Fabulous. I couldn't wish for a better moment.

'Why have you got a pornographic picture of yourself on this computer?' my mum asked, getting straight to the point.

I got defensive, 'It's not pornographic, it's my arse! Just a bum. See! It's harmless, a bit of fun. It's not like you can see my face!'

My mum looked at me, her own face going crimson.

'I hope you're not using it on one of those sites to … you know … get men,' my dad stuttered.

'Nope, I'm not,' I grinned at my mum, 'at least … not any more.'

My mum grinned back, and for a moment I'm sure she

beamed at me, with what seemed like a little pride. Here was her daughter, brought up to respect her own sexuality and be proud of her desires and wants, being her own woman and keeping up the good work she'd fought and struggled for in the Sixties. When she smiled at me I felt she understood me; it was a brief but powerful moment between us.

My dad, however, was po-faced and silent. Then he stood up and started to walk out, my mum following closely behind. 'Perhaps you might want to get rid of it?' he said, as they left the room.

I immediately sat down and deleted the photo, then searched through his entire computer to see if there were any other remnants I might have left behind. Thank God there were none. At least, I couldn't find any pictures of erect cocks; maybe I was more careful in those days than I recall. So the damage limitation was minor: my shame survived to live another day.

So my parents know a little too much about me now, more than I wanted them to. It's not that they are at all prudish or old-fashioned, or even disapprove of me having a sexually active lifestyle – the opposite in fact. But having the evidence thrust in their faces leaves me, and I am sure them too, feeling uncomfortable.

But it's reminded me just how good in bed Karl is and I'm looking forward to meeting him on Friday – and finally getting another good seeing to.

Friday 30th September

It wasn't until I was sitting on Karl's face that I began to cry.

Up until then I thought I was alright, but my sensitivity

was heightened by the powerful orgasm he'd induced with his tongue and my brain finally kicked into gear. I was overcome by all the emotion I had been holding back.

Karl and I had a lot to catch up on. Our lives now are as disparate as the distance between us. I couldn't wait to see him, and, of course, rip his clothes off and fuck him all night. What better way to get Blog Boy out of my head, I thought, than to de-fuck myself of him, with someone else?

But when, after much vodka, Karl gently pressed his mouth to mine and kissed me deeply it felt wrong somehow, though I just put it down to my drunkenness and ignored it, pulling him close so I could feel his hardness against me. I concentrated on the delicious throbbing sensation between my legs.

After pulling off my underwear and kissing me all over, Karl lowered himself down my body, his tongue lightly dabbing and flicking while his fingers gently caressed me. I watched him for a moment, and something slowly began to dawn on me.

I didn't want to be with him.

Not because he wasn't turning me on – he was – but because he was not the person I wanted to turn me on. I wanted it to be Blog Boy.

I thought that by now I would have been able to accept that Blog Boy didn't want anything serious with me. I thought I was doing OK. But now it struck me that perhaps I wasn't coping as well as I previously thought; for the first time in my life, I was having sex with someone and imagining I was with somebody else. As Karl slipped his fingers inside me, I thought of how much Blog Boy turned me on; as my orgasm hit, I recalled his face smiling at me, and it made me climax even harder.

Then I looked down at Karl and felt guilty.

I pushed him off me, and threw him onto his back. At least if I gave him some pleasure, all would be well, I thought. And having had sex with him many times over the years, I am familiar with his preferences: I immediately lowered my mouth to his perineum and slid both my hands around his shaft before sucking his cock deeply.

He responded well and ground his hips into my face within moments, but soon it became apparent that something was wrong. Or, more specifically, something was wrong with me. I wasn't enjoying giving Karl a blow job. I was trying to pleasure him, but it wasn't his cock that I wanted in my mouth, it was Blog Boy's.

I looked up at Karl and I knew that it was pointless to continue. It was feeling like a chore, not a pleasure, and I know he was picking up that vibe from me. His penis was getting softer by the minute which was totally out of character.

Karl pulled me up over him and begged me to do his favourite thing: sit on his face. Not really my preference, but at that point, two orgasms in, I felt obliged to do something he would enjoy. So I crouched over him and lowered myself onto his waiting, eager tongue.

With each lick he gave me, I felt sadder. With each nibble he offered, I felt guiltier. As his tongue lapped away enthusiastically and I felt the waves of pleasure emanating from my body, I was filled with self-hatred. How could I just use him like that? Was I really such a sex fiend that I could allow myself to be physically pleasured by someone even though I didn't want to be with them? With these thoughts I felt my horniness dissipate, and I frantically concentrated on the sensations between my legs, knowing that I was nearing climax and I so badly needed the release – if only to let go of the emotional tension building up inside of me.

I closed my eyes and gripped the bed frame, and as my orgasm approached, a thought suddenly entered my head: Blog Boy didn't want me, and no matter how much I liked him, nothing would come of it. With my body shaking, I saw his face in my mind, felt the tears stream down my cheeks, and I gritted my teeth to bear both the intensity of the climax and the intensity of my emotions.

After a few minutes, when my spasms subsided, Karl cuddled up to me, and placed his hard cock in my hand. I looked at him and at his cock, and knew I couldn't do it. I pulled my hand away. 'I'm sorry; I'm not really with it tonight.'

'What's up?'

'This guy ... my head is a bit all over the place ...'

'A recent break-up?'

'Not really: we didn't even go out together. I am just a stupid twat.'

'Why?'

'It's not requited.'

'Oh, I'm sorry. That's tough.'

'Stupid, more like.'

'Don't be so hard on yourself, these things happen.'

'Yeah, well, I was fully aware from the start that he didn't want to get involved, so I have no excuse for feeling crap.'

'It happens to the best of us.'

'I guess. Anyway, I did all this' – I gestured at our mutual nakedness – 'to realise just how much I liked him. I'm sorry; I didn't mean to ruin your evening.'

'Don't worry about it. Sometimes it happens, sometimes it doesn't; you know that. It's no big deal, relax.'

'Sorry all the same; I thought I was fine up until now.'

'It's OK. So you on speaking terms?'

'Not really – the last time we spoke was when we slept together, and that was more than a month ago. I guess he's been trying to avoid me. He's away travelling now. I doubt he'll contact me.'

'Us men can be a bit crap sometimes.'

'Well, it's my own fault, always picking ones who are unattainable. Anyway ... onward and upward and all that.'

'That's the spirit. Someone else will come along.'

'Yup; let's hope.'

And with that Karl switched out the light and spooned me, wrapping his arms around my waist and sliding his thighs underneath mine. He kissed my back and neck gently and then drifted off to sleep.

I know his holding me was Karl's way of being affectionate and he probably thought it was what I wanted and he was right, I did want to be held – just not by him. Instead it reminded me of what I really wanted – *who* I really wanted – and that Blog Boy didn't want that with me.

As soon as Karl fell asleep, I moved out of his embrace. I lay there for hours, unable to sleep, the constant hum of traffic and Karl's rhythmic snoring filling the room with white noise, adding to the loudness of the thoughts in my own head. I knew it was irrational to think it, but in my highly emotional and drunken state, I began to wonder that perhaps if I was prettier, or less of a sex fiend, or less neurotic, maybe then Blog Boy would want to be with me.

And I lay there and thought about why I was single, why the men I fall for don't seem to fall for me, and why I was having meaningless sex with someone I didn't care about, when two months ago I had been having sex with someone I did.

I knew I had to get out of there and collect my thoughts. I wanted to be on my own, not curled up with this man. When the dawn broke and the first rays of light streamed into the room, I quietly got out of bed, put on my clothes and made my way to the door.

I turned as I reached it, and looked back. Karl was still asleep. Even though my impulse was to leave immediately, I felt he deserved more than that. After all, we've been fuck-buddies for many years and I value and respect him.

So I woke him up and apologised, explaining that I needed to be on my own. Thankfully he was sympathetic, and kissed me on the forehead before wishing me well and sending me on my way.

I left the flat, walked through the estate, jumped onto the tube with the early morning commuters, and, as I found a place to sit, felt tears silently rolling down my cheeks, and my make-up smearing under my sunglasses.

As I wept on the journey home today, it struck me just how empty casual sex can feel – how difficult it can be when you want more, or have feelings for someone else. And it made me realise that sometimes even orgasms induced by another can feel lonely.

The Girl's Guide to Why Men Should Shave Their Genitals

1 It can make a cock look bigger

2 It makes the area appear neater and well groomed

3 Women are more likely to get stuck in if it looks like a bloke takes care of his genitals

4 Removing the hair means there's less sweat in the area

5 The cock and balls will smell fresher

6 The cock and balls will taste fresher

7 The cock and balls will feel nicer in a lover's mouth without the barrier of hair

8 Fewer hairs will end up in a lover's mouth

9 There will be an increase in sensation for the man when he has a tongue wrapped around his cock

10 If women can go through the pain and tedium of shaving, waxing and plucking their nether regions, so can bloody men

10

October

Saturday 1st October

I decided to go for a long run in my local park today to try to clear my head. I feel a bit confused about things right now; what happened with Karl has thrown me a little. I've never been upset by a good, honest shag before – I feel like the world as I know it is upside down.

So I did six miles and I feel much better for it now. I was on the phone to Kathy a minute ago, bragging about my running speed, and she asked me what I think about when I train, to help me stay focussed. I was very tempted to say 'cock', though of course I didn't.

It *is* the truth, but I doubt very much that she would be able to cope with my honesty, since she has, when I have responded similarly sexually in the past, retorted, 'Oh my God, Abby, you are obsessed!' and then quickly changed the subject, shifting uncomfortably in her seat.

So, instead of telling her what was really going through my mind, I made it up:

a) the end objective – how good I will feel when I have finished running the distance

b) pushing myself to 'go just five more minutes', then

'another five minutes', and then 'C'mon, Abby, what's another twenty minutes on top of that?'

c) getting myself into a 'zone', where I feel peaceful, calm and focussed on my breathing

d) recalling how my ex, Steven, pissed me off, and remembering what a wanker he was, gritting my teeth and running even faster

e) thinking how gutted he would be to see me now, as I tone my thighs and arse even more

f) listening to Maximo Park and knowing that I can beat the timing of the guitar riff in 'Apply Some Pressure', now that I have overcome that bastard hill

g) looking at the park/street/road I am running on, and acknowledging that London can in fact be a beautiful city to live in

h) feeling the endorphins flowing through my body as I sprint for the last five minutes of the hour

Well, I'm not technically lying to Kathy, just not telling her the whole truth. If I had answered her *truthfully*, what could I have possibly said?

a) that when I ran past that handsome blond man, I knew he was looking at my erect nipples, and as I imagined his hands slipping off my top to free my breasts, it helped me run faster?

b) that as I got to the brow of the hill, I saw two guys walking towards me, and the vision I had of me between them, one cock in each hand, sucking them alternately, made me sprint to the top and race down the other side?

c) that when I saw a woman wearing a body-hugging wrap-dress and no knickers, I wanted to lift her skirt up and slide my hands between her legs, and this thought made me sprint past her and race alongside the traffic on the road?

d) that if I concentrate on recalling the sex I last had with Blog Boy in detail, then before I know it ten minutes have passed and I am nearer my end objective?

e) that if I think about Jamie and concentrate on what it would feel like to have his cock in my mouth, his fingers between my legs, then his cock pummelling me, then a good 20 minutes fly by and I get closer to my end objective?

f) that when I listen to Maximo Park, and it gets to the guitar riff in 'Apply Some Pressure', I think about how nice it would be to listen to the song when I was on my hands and knees, getting fucked hard from behind. With this thought, overcoming hills is no obstacle.

g) that if I see a couple making out in the park, I wonder whether the girl would be circling the outline of her lover's cock with her thumb like I would, and the tingle that this thought gives me spurs me on even faster?

h) that with a constant throbbing and wetness between my legs whilst I run, the pulse of my clit feels like an extra heartbeat pushing the blood round my body and energises me, forcing me to work harder?

The reality is that no matter how many times I might have a quick frig before a run, I always get turned on when I'm exercising, so instead of being preoccupied with the things normal runners think about (targets, breathing, muscle cramp), I'm thinking about what is happening between my legs.

And this makes me want to play again. So I figure that the

harder I run, the quicker I can finish, and finally reward my pussy with another workout.

Sadly, I don't think Kathy could ever deal with all this. It's one thing being an anonymous sex fiend writing a diary, but it's quite another to have your mates thinking that you are always gagging for a shag.

Even if it is true.

Sunday 2nd October

Maybe I ran too hard yesterday, or perhaps it's just period pain, but today my legs are sore and I am aching all over.

I can't wait to finish my period and be done with it. At least then I'll be completely free of pain and able to run with ease, not to mention, most importantly, that then I'll be free to shag without worrying about leaking blood everywhere.

This has happened to every woman, I am sure. There's always that final dreg of blood to our period – a last gush that always, without fail, ruins our favourite knickers, or during shagging, bathes some poor bloke in enough gore to make it look like he's been in a battle, not a bed. Not a pleasant situation. I've even had that final spurt when Karl was eating my pussy some years ago:

'I thought you tasted metallic,' he said to me later, as I groaned with embarrassment and felt obliged to give him a blow job for an hour to make up for covering his stomach and cock with what seemed like gallons of blood.

But when the same thing happened with Steven last year, I was actually pleased.

We were fucking on his couch by candlelight. He was

exploring every inch of my body with his hands; thrusting his fingers in and out of me, making me climax over and over again.

I remember feeling extra slippery, as though I was really gushing every time I came, more even than my usual miniature waterfall ... And as it turned out, I was.

I had climaxed six or seven times before he finally gave me what I wanted: his cock. He fucked me hard. He took me from on top, underneath, side by side, behind, and finally – my ankles around his neck – kneeling in front of me, grinding into me, making us both climax together intensely.

Drunk and tired, we went straight to bed afterwards and immediately fell asleep.

When I got up to make some coffee the next morning, I got a fright. For a moment I thought an intruder had broken into the flat and killed someone. There was blood everywhere. Not just specks or spots but scarlet handprints all over the couch, like the aftermath of some act of despicable violence.

I looked at them and retraced the events of the night before, like a forensic scientist after a murder: ah yes, that was where he had me on all fours and was trying to fist me. Oh, that must have been the moment when I sat on top of him and he was rubbing my g-spot, and oh yes, that was when I was on the edge of the couch and he was ramming his cock into me as fast as he could.

For a moment, I felt dreadfully guilty. I had thought my period was over and hadn't expected the bleeding, but it was *my* blood after all, and his pale cream couch was ruined. But then I got over it.

I'm not a vindictive or malicious person who holds grudges, but somehow, given that he was cheating on me – it seemed like some kind of karmic retribution. My body had found a way to royally shaft him. It was better than telephoning him and hanging up; more effective than cutting up his clothes; more original than letting down his car tyres – by bleeding all over his precious couch, my body was telling Steven: 'Fuck you, you prick.'

It felt good.

And when I went back for one last fuck, a month later, this utterly house-proud man still hadn't managed to get all my blood out of the fabric.

I was very sad when I finally walked away from that situation, but that little bit of sadistic pleasure I got from knowing that I'd left my mark on his world more than made up for the heartbreak.

Saturday 8th October

Jamie and I met up again last night. I knew my instincts were right – there's definitely an attraction between us – and just ten minutes into the evening we were flirting openly with each other. I was relieved that we were; I need a mental – and a physical – distraction from Blog Boy, after all.

We kept touching each other, a hand on an arm here, a quick touch there, so it was inevitable that we would end up snogging, and we did, passionately.

An hour of long, slow snogging later, Jamie said to me, 'I want you to do something for me when you go to the toilet.'

I was confused but tried to cover it, smiling. 'What is it that you want me to do?'

He leant in towards me and said softly, 'I want you to

put your finger inside yourself, so I can taste you when you come back.'

My pussy tingled with excitement. I thought about what he had asked and took a deep breath, before shyly replying, 'I think that can be arranged.'

He smiled at me, and I grinned back, kissed him once more and then made my way to the loo.

I'd been dying for a piss for the last half-hour, but I found myself in some difficulty. My pussy was so swollen that it was practically impossible to urinate.

So, this is what it's like trying to pee with an erection, I thought to myself, as I focussed on attempting to squeeze out even the smallest bit of urine. My clit was so engorged it was like a miniature hard-on.

But eventually – some minutes later – I managed it, and set to work on the task in, er, hand.

It was the first time I had received such a request, so I wondered what the procedure should be:

★ Which finger should I use? Should it be more than one?
★ Is it right to fully insert it, or should I just rub it against my soaked vulva?
★ How wet should the finger be? Knuckle-deep in juice? Or just an elegantly moist fingertip?

Questions, questions.

I rubbed myself absentmindedly as I pondered these problems, knowing that he would shortly be tasting me and discovering how turned on I was.

I was sharply snapped out of this delightful fantasy when someone hammered on the toilet door and demanded that I hurry up. I quickly slipped my middle finger deep inside myself, soaked it in my juices, and made my way back to Jamie.

As I approached him, it suddenly struck me that there was even more to the correct etiquette for this little interaction. Was I supposed to just hold out my finger to him, and say:

'Here you go, fresh pussy juice for you?'

Or perhaps, slide my finger under his nose, and ask:

'Like the smell?'

Or maybe, just show him my wet finger and then wipe the juice off on something?

Why isn't there a rule book for these things? How was a well-brought-up girl like me supposed to offer a finger covered in her own pussy juice to a guy she barely knew? What was the acceptable and polite procedure?

I felt so 'English' as I made my way through the crowded bar that for all my recent sex-fiendishness I still felt uncomfortable and embarrassed.

There was no need. He smiled at me as I got near and began to kiss me as soon as I sat down next to him. And as our kiss got deeper and more passionate, I lifted my hand to his face, and slowly wiped my wet finger across his lips. Finding the tip of it with his tongue, he pulled it into his mouth and began to suck hard.

Feeling his hot mouth devouring my juices made me want him even more and, with my finger sliding between our mouths, I kissed him deeply, tasting myself on his lips as I did so.

It turned me on so much … and when he whispered in my ear, 'You taste delicious,' I wanted to tug down his trousers, pull down his pants and draw his cock into my mouth and tell him exactly the same thing.

Trouble was, we were in a well-lit, crowded bar, and I very much doubt that displaying genitalia or participating in public sex acts would have been considered acceptable behaviour there.

As we sat there, he began to stroke my arse and said softly in my ear, 'You weren't lying earlier.'

'About what?'

'About not wearing any underwear,' he replied, running his hand along the curve of my bum where my knickers would have been, had I chosen to wear them.

'I would never lie about something as important as that,' I said. 'Anyway, I just forgot to put them on.'

He laughed, 'Of course, that must be it – you forgot.'

I grinned cheekily at him, and felt his hand travel lower down my arse cheek. Moving my arm to stabilise myself, I placed my hand on the couch between his legs, and noticed that if I subtly rested my forearm against him I could feel his stiffening cock pushed up against me through his jeans.

'Mmm', he said, his knob giving a little twitch against my arm, 'that feels good.'

I pushed my arm further back and could now feel his cock straining behind the denim. His hand gently tugged at my dress; his fingers exploring my bare skin under it.

I looked at him smiling at me, felt the throbbing between my legs increase tenfold, and tried to think clearly. We were sitting in a public bar. There were people sitting either side of us on the couch. To indulge in any more of this sort of play surely meant attracting attention to ourselves and that was appealing in itself, but this was not really the right environment in which to explore my newly found exhibitionist tendencies.

I barely knew Jamie and had been trying to maintain

dignified intellectual conversation with him, and I was worried that if I indulged my carnal desires like I did with Blog Boy, it might scupper the possibility of something other than sex developing between us.

The main problem, though, was that I was all too aware of the fact that my pussy was fucking soaking and I was immensely turned on and needed some release. Feeling his erection pressed up against the back of my forearm was driving me crazy. All I wanted to do was zip open his trousers and grip his cock in my hands, and for his fingers to slide further down so he could discover how wet I was.

I tried desperately hard to focus – to remind myself that I was not a slave to my lust, and that I could be dignified and friendly and manage to make a connection on a non-sexual level. I could behave myself in public, even with a dripping wet pussy.

As he carried on regardless, gently stroking my arse, I couldn't bear it any more, and I raised myself so he could slide his fingers under my dress and down between my legs. Then I sat on his hand.

'My God, you're wet,' he murmured in my ear, as he rubbed his fingers along my pussy.

Jesus, it felt good: too good. As he stroked me lightly, I felt myself quiver, and I couldn't stop myself from gently shifting on his hand and asking him to put his fingers inside me.

Waves of pleasure washed over me as his fingers entered me; I responded the only way I could in this very public place, pushing my forearm back and forth in time against his substantial trouser-bulge.

It all felt divine: his fingers softly stroking my wetness, my arm pressing against his erection. I was getting carried away by it all, my pleasure increasing with each stroke he gave me and each pulse of his cock against my forearm.

And then I knew what was to come. That is – me coming. It was inevitable, there was nothing I could do to stop it. Forget men and their 'point of no return': there are no brakes that can stop *my* orgasm train. I glanced to the left and saw my neighbours deep in conversation, and then I grabbed the edge of the couch and steeled myself in an effort to make my shuddering less noticeable.

Feeling his fingers moving faster inside me, it was all I could do to stop myself shouting, 'Oh God, fuck me, I need you to fuck me!', unzipping him and climbing onto his cock to sit reverse-cowgirl and ride him hard.

I had to hold my breath, grit my teeth, and feel my body and all my muscles become rigid as I held back the shaking and convulsions. I came violently, dripping onto his fingers.

'You're so naughty,' he breathed in my ear, kissing my neck.

Still shaking from the aftershocks, I said breathlessly, 'It's you! You're bringing it out of me.'

He laughed, and kept moving his fingers inside me – a dangerous thing to do, especially when I then promptly had three more orgasms as he went on fingering me in clear view of at least 70 other people. It should have been some cause of concern for me, but I'm amazed to say it wasn't.

Preoccupied with his hand constantly moving between my legs, I concentrated on the sensations in my pussy and the answering throb of his cock pushing up against my forearm, and somehow all my worries and inhibitions disappeared.

When a mutual acquaintance came over to our couch to say goodbye to everyone on it, I whispered to Jamie, 'What if he reaches out to shake your hand?' He grinned at me, and rubbed me harder, replying, 'I was thinking the exact same thought.'

With the fingers of his right hand fully engaged, and my thumb now circling the outline of his cock through his jeans, we politely waited to bid our farewells. Luckily, this didn't include a handshake and Jamie's fingers were still sunk deep into me when the friend made his way round to us to wish us well for the night.

'I'm not sure I can take much more of this,' I said, after he'd gone.

Jamie moaned as his cock stiffened against my touch and looked at me, the frustration clear in his eyes. I had been a little cruel. It wasn't intentional, but given the circumstances, and my female physiology, it was far easier for him covertly to push his fingers inside me, than it was for me to have my hand around his cock.

So instead, I surreptitiously hid my hand underneath his shirt and rubbed his swollen cock through his jeans with my fingers. He groaned again, and I felt the heat of it through the thick denim.

'God, your cock is hard,' I remarked, slightly shocked by the response I was getting from the light touch I was giving him. 'I don't know how much more I can take of this; I just want to take it out now and hold it.'

He responded by sliding his fingers further inside me again, making me shiver and shake once more.

'Fuck, I can't bear this,' I said, as I pressed my palm down, 'I want your cock inside me now!'

'I want to be inside you too.' He gave me a long kiss, and as his tongue danced in my mouth, I tried to think.

OK, so I had already crossed the friendship barrier with

Jamie. It was too late to pretend otherwise. Surely it could do no harm to go further? It would give me what I'd been craving all night. There was no turning back. I had to fuck him – and fast.

I leaned over to him and whispered, 'Are you thinking what I'm thinking?'

'The lavatory?'

'Yes. We've both got condoms with us, after all.'

He grinned. I continued, somewhat excitedly: 'You could follow me in and have a seat on the toilet. I could just lift my dress and then sit on your cock. How does that sound?'

'I'm not going to be able to last long,' he warned me, 'not after all this.' He motioned to my thumb, still busy in his lap.

'Neither am I,' I pressed down harder, 'but I need to feel your cock inside me.'

He nodded, wincing, 'Sounds good to me.'

He removed his hand from my crotch as I started to get up. 'You do know you are going to leave a huge wet patch on the seat, don't you?' he joked.

'Fuck it, it's leather, no one will notice,' I responded, somewhat unconvincingly, worried I'd turn to see a small puddle of liquid on the seat, glinting under the ceiling lights.

'Your dress is fine,' he said, as I tried to adjust it, and at the time I believed him, so I walked straight into the toilet.

He followed me in and within moments we were locked in the cubicle, his hands freeing my breasts from my dress and bra, my hands tearing down his jeans to get to his penis.

There was barely enough room in there for one person to stand, let alone for two people to fuck, but we managed it. As he entered me I heard him grunt, and I felt my orgasm build and increase in its intensity; the moment he released his, I let go, clutching at him as I came like a fucking train.

237

We sat there, sweaty, shaking and laughing, finally released from the pent-up horniness. But then he started to play with my nipples and set me off again, and I came hard once more.

'Sorry about that,' I said, 'you started me up again. I knew there was one more waiting to come out. Six orgasms in one night – I think I owe you! Perhaps we should try this again sometime to even out the score a bit – maybe somewhere a little more spacious?'

He agreed and laughed and kissed me once more, and I felt happy and excited that he wanted to see me again. Perhaps I could finally put Blog Boy behind me now.

After a little while I stood up and we fixed our clothing and left the bar. Saying goodnight, I made my way to my night bus.

It was only when I sat down that I realised just how wrong he had been about my dress. Not only was it absolutely sopping, but when I looked at it later I discovered my come all over it too.

Not a bad thing, but it certainly explained all the stares I got from people as I made my way home.

Wednesday 12th October

One of the things that most attracts me to men is their brain. I know I wrote that I loved a tall man with big hands, but what really gets me going is a man's ability to express himself intellectually. The biggest aphrodisiac of all is intelligence.

After meeting Blog Boy and Jamie, I am becoming aware that I find it simultaneously attractive and intimidating to be in the company of a man whom I find intellectually challenging. I love the fact that they can stimulate my mind and fire up my neurons, but I also feel nervous faced with the possibility that they'll highlight my own intellectual weaknesses. The result of this paradox is excitement. Ergo, I feel aroused.

Thinking about this reminds me of one of my tutors at college years ago. A few years older than me, he was not a particularly attractive man. He drank and smoked far too much and obviously indulged in unhealthy eating – he was pretty out of shape. He had no dress sense and it was clear that he was quite a geek – not exactly the testosterone-fuelled Alpha Male that women are supposed to go weak at the knees for.

Yet I am sure he had pussy falling out of his pockets.

Or at least he would have had my pussy falling out of his pocket had I decided to cross the line between tutor and student.

You see, regardless of how he looked or carried himself, the man had a brain on him, and that was intolerably sexy to me. My mind would go to mush every time he talked about Postmodernism. One mention of Derrida, and I was captivated. A brief exploration of Lyotard and I was hooked. A quick attack on McLuhan and my heart started beating faster. When he told us pornography was a transgressive movement against conservatism, I was smitten.

It is fair to say that I had a massive crush on his mind.

During his lectures, I would sit there, transfixed by his arguments, his every word making my breath race and my pussy tighten. On more than one occasion, I would have to leave the lecture hall to go to the toilet to relieve myself. I even sat at the back of the room so that I could make a quick exit for my frig. For three years.

And after the lectures, we would have seminars – otherwise known as getting drunk with the tutors in the cheap student bar. We got on very well of course, and would spend hours in debate, discussion, or in blazing arguments, seeing who could down the most beers at the same time. Other students would join us, but the connection between us two was on another level. And that level was sex.

He read me very well. Not only because I regularly wrote theses about feminism, pornography and sexuality, but through our discussions about sex, and our ability to be totally frank with each other, I knew that he was as open-minded as me – if not more so. Not many students would know that their tutor liked to tie his partners up, and whip, spank and tease them, before fucking them hard, but I knew this – and more – about him.

Despite that, neither of us explored the sexual tension that swirled around us. Apart from the fact that student/teacher relationships were strictly forbidden, I didn't want anything to jeopardise my studies.

I was hungry for knowledge and a proud student too. I absorbed every piece of information I could and I always strived to be the best. I would get disappointed if I got less than an A minus in any subject, and would work even harder to ensure that my grades kept up to the A pluses I expected of myself. If I had fucked my tutor it would have meant that I couldn't trust his marking: something I couldn't bear to have happen. I wanted to know that I had earned and deserved every mark I got and not to have to worry that he was swayed by my sexual ability.

So we didn't shag and I'm thankful, because it meant I knew my final mark was based on my knowledge, hard work and ability to construct a killer argument – skills I have tried to maintain in my everyday adult life.

And, of course, not fucking him left me wanting more. I learned that there is nothing nicer than being on the edge of your chair with excitement in a debate with someone who you find intellectually stimulating – especially if your body is fully engaged too.

So I am very much looking forward to seeing Jamie again. I'd like to revisit the rough and ready, downright horny sex, but I hope I'll get a little bit more than that too – a brain fuck into the bargain.

Tuesday 18th October

Yesterday I had a conversation with a work colleague called Pete about the number of sexual partners we have each enjoyed. I suspected my tally would be far higher than his, and the conversation seemed to be running along on two levels.

'How many men have you slept with, then?' Pete asked. *I want to find out how experienced/slutty you are.*

'You know a lady can never divulge such things,' I replied. 'It's a woman's right to keep her exact age, her weight and the number of lovers she's had to herself.' *Which of course is a load of fucking bollocks, and I would gladly tell you the answers to all three if I weren't so sure that you'd judge me on the last one.*

'Oh, come on, I won't judge you. I'm just curious. It's no big deal, however many it might be.' *Except that it can't possibly be more women than I have slept with, since that would leave me feeling insecure about my own sexual prowess.*

'If it's not a big deal, then I'm not going to tell you. Some things are best kept personal.' *If you knew how many, you would stop chatting me up instantly.*

'Look, it really doesn't matter to me. I'm just wondering.

If it's a lot, I don't have a problem with that. It just means you're more skilled than most, which isn't a bad thing.' *I hope it's not a lot.*

'Seriously, I'm not going to tell you; guys always pass judgment on women based on how many people they've fucked, even if they say they don't.' *And the hypocritical double-standard about what is considered acceptable for men, as opposed to women, pisses me off.*

'I won't. I tell you what, I'll write down how many women I have slept with on a bit of paper and then you can tell me whether your number is higher or lower.' *And that way I can write whatever I think is a large number, so that you think I have a lot of experience.*

He jotted down something onto a scrap of paper and handed it to me, ensuring his fingers lingered on mine as he dropped the note into my hand. I opened the note up and smiled. *Bet he exaggerated the number to impress me. Boy, would he be shocked with my number. Fuck it, maybe I should just tell him.*

'So, what is it, then?' Pete asked. *Let's hope it's below that figure. Please, let it be below that figure.*

I paused for a moment. 'Let's just say that with me, you could double that figure.' *Actually you could triple it or even quadruple it, and you'd still be quite a few off.*

'Really?' Pete exclaimed. 'Wow. I mean, hey – that's great, each to their own, some people are more experienced than others, right? That's wonderful.' *What a slut. There's no way I could date her knowing that. Glad I found that out now.*

'Yup. Anyway, I've found it's irrelevant how many lovers a person has had; for me it's all about someone's enthusiasm, interest and open-mindedness, not to mention there being a great mental connection – that's what makes great sex.'

Alongside an ability not to judge, which clearly, looking at the stunned expression on your face, you are having a hard time doing right now.

'I agree. Oops, I really should get back to the set; it's been fun chatting.' *But I don't think this situation will be developing any further now.*

'It's been fun, yeah. And nice to know that there are some open-minded men out there.' *Shame you're not one of them.*

He kissed me on the cheek and wandered off, leaving me standing there clutching the piece of paper in my hand.

What a twat. I'm beginning to give up hope on men.

Wednesday 19th October

I'm still fuming from that conversation with Pete. Why judge someone's attractiveness by the number of sexual partners that they've had? Why should it matter? It does, clearly. In my own experience – which is obviously too much for Pete to deal with – men have three different ways of behaving when confronted by a woman who's had a lot of lovers:

1) **The intimidated man.** Although perhaps turned on by the woman's sexual confidence, these men are essentially put off by her sexual history, because they find it daunting that she might have more experience – for this, read better skills – in bed than them.

   They might want to be the one with all the sex-tricks, not the one *learning* them. They worry that they won't be able to satisfy her in bed, so they back away from exploring any intimacy with her, both physical and mental. That's not to say they don't frantically masturbate when thinking about her, though.

2) **The confident man**. These men are not intimidated. Rather they are turned on by the knowledge. They equate this with a high sex drive and assume that they are then almost guaranteed a good fuck with her. They still feel relaxed about their own sexual expertise, too.

On the down side, the fact that they are driven by their focus on shagging her, rather than connecting with her mentally, means they may not achieve any intimacy with her. Also, since their expectations of her sexual prowess might be unrealistic, they will quite possibly end up being disappointed, when the reality doesn't match their fantasy. Again, some frantic masturbating is involved, but it usually occurs prior to the sex and rarely continues after it.

3) **The man who wants to 'tame' a woman.** These men are neither put off nor highly turned on by the woman's previous sexual history. Instead, their challenge is to try to make the woman become monogamous – and monogamous with *them* – thus proving that their own sexual prowess was enough to make the woman 'settle down'.

Again, their expectations might be unrealistic: if a woman is in no hurry to enter a long-term relationship, then no amount of devotion to her pussy will make her give up her lifestyle. I am assuming some regular masturbating occurs for the male in question here too, but most likely involves the addition of the mental image of a white picket fence and a dog.

In my experience, most men I've met fall into group one when faced with a sexually confident/experienced woman. Next in line are the number two's, and lastly the number three's who are few in number and I've only bumped into them a couple of times.

I have nothing against any of the men I have described – in fact I have occasionally, wistfully wished that a few more number one's would give me a chance, but I am still hoping that a man will one day say to me:

'How many partners? I really don't care actually. Let's just get to know each other, and see if we have a connection, OK?'

Jamie seems to be the latter. I hope so, anyway.

Friday 21st October

Just got an email from Jamie. I opened it eagerly but couldn't believe my eyes when I read what he had written.

He's got back together with his ex. He won't be able to meet up with me again.

I can't say I'm not disappointed – I am. Massively gutted, actually.

Though we only met twice, given the scores of emails and text messages we sent and the fantastic sex we had, I felt like we had a great connection. It was reassuring that he was so open about sex too; finally, I thought, here's a man who is on my level and will understand my obsession.

So it's all over now and I suppose I just have to believe that it wasn't meant to be. Why do I have such bad luck with blokes?

By a weird coincidence Blog Boy has emailed me too – finally. He said he was really looking forward to seeing me again when he gets back from his travels in a couple of weeks. He apologised profusely for the drop in communication before he went away, saying he was very stressed out with work and trying to sort the trip and that he hoped he hadn't offended me by not being in touch.

I am trying not to read anything into it. He's probably just feeling homesick right now, but I *am* pleased that he contacted me. And I'm glad he reiterated the fact that he still wants to be friends with me – hopefully, he means it.

Though of course I'd be lying if I said I still didn't want more with him.

Thursday 27th October

With how things turned out with Blog Boy and now Jamie, I've decided to go to New York once again to have some time away from the men here in London. They're just confusing me.

There's not much work around and I've got some time on my hands. I need to do something positive and get out of town.

So I'm off in a few days, staying with Harry once more. I can't wait to see him and tell him about all my adventures this year.

Perhaps I'll even have some more fun when I'm in the States. Here's hoping.

The Girl's Guide to Qualities Sought in a Man

The basic	Preferred	Ideal	Unrealistic, but one can always hope
Single	Single, never been married	Single, never been married, no kids, has lots of female and gay friends	Only spends 10 per cent of his 'alone' time wanking to girl-on-girl porn
Intelligent	Educated	Worldly	Good in bed
Non-sexist	Knows that *Nuts* magazine is porn pretending to be entertainment	Agrees how unfair it is that most porn is made solely from the male perspective	Actively seeks out feminist female-made porn for you
Left wing	Pacifist and non-violent	Green: does his bit for the environment	Happy to carry your bags when you go on demos
Likes animals	Is gentle with animals when handling them (note: future baby handling)	Is compassionate about animals' welfare	Won't take you to KFC for dinner
Eats healthily	His diet isn't limited to a kilo of red meat per day	Enjoys cooking	Doesn't spend three hours 'reading' Nigella Lawson
Isn't an alcoholic	Occasionally drinks	Likes a good wine rather than a beer with a meal	Won't go out every Friday with his mates and get slaughtered

The basic	Preferred	Ideal	Unrealistic, but one can always hope
Kind	Thoughtful	Generous	Remembers your birthday
Affectionate and tactile	Gives you lots of hugs	Shows you affection in public	Touches you in non-sexual ways too
Loving and sensitive	Able to give emotional support	Able to receive emotional support	Able to talk about his feelings without having to be drunk
Honest and trustworthy	Can trust him with all your darkest secrets	Will tell you when your arse looks big	Will never show anyone the naked pictures he took of you
Wants to be in a relationship	Wants to be in a long-term relationship	Wants to be in a long-term relationship with you alone	Wants kids
Not threatened by an assertive woman	Similarly assertive	Able to express his sexual and emotional needs	Will not expect you to dress up in rubber and whip him senseless on a nightly basis
Open-minded	Sexually adventurous	Wants to explore your and his sexual fantasies	Can also fuck in missionary position
Good sex drive	High sex drive	Rampant sex drive	Always up for it

11

November

Wednesday 2nd November

As soon as I got through Customs I knew I would see him.

Not that there was any logic to that gut feeling, but as I turned the corner I felt his presence and sure enough there he was, standing by the far wall.

Nick had aged quite a bit since I last saw him. His dark hair is now a mass of grey curls and his face is etched with more lines than I remembered. He looked more handsome than ever; his beautiful eyes lit up when he caught sight of me and the laughter lines around them set off his wide smile.

'Oh, my God! Abby! I don't believe it!' he exclaimed, and walked towards me, arms outstretched.

He embraced me tightly, making my spine tingle as he touched the bare skin under the straps of my tank top. I felt the muscles on his back flex as I wrapped my arms around him and remembered how much I used to adore his strong shoulders, how I used to trace them with my fingertips before pressing my breasts against them.

As we hugged and I rested my head on him, I caught the freshness of his smell. I had an impulse to kiss his neck gently, as I used to, but instead I inhaled deeply – as if to preserve the scent-memory of him – and squeezed him tighter.

We pulled back and did the embarrassing dance of two English people who have previously been intimate – where should we kiss each other hello? We finally settled – somewhat haphazardly – on each other's cheek, as awkward as teenagers.

'What are you doing here?' he asked, looking thrilled.

'I'm staying with some friends and also meeting up with my folks when they're in town,' I said. 'Hopefully I'll still be sane at the end of it, but I doubt it.'

He laughed and the lines around his eyes crinkled warmly. I remembered being seduced by those same eyes, that and his wit, charm and northern accent.

'What about you?' I asked. 'You on holiday too?'

'No, I live here now,' he replied. 'I've been stuck here for the last hour waiting for a friend to arrive.' He gestured at the Arrivals board above my head.

'Oh, wow. I didn't know you'd moved.' I was shocked that I hadn't known something so major. It suddenly seemed like an age since our lives were synchronised, a lifetime since he lay next to me, stroking the hair away from my eyes.

'So, you still doing music stuff, then?' I asked.

'Yep, bits and bobs. Mostly writing for others now.'

I recalled how the broken-heartedness of his lyrics showed a more gentle side to his otherwise rugged, laddish exterior. The first time I watched him perform the melancholic melodies his skilful guitar-playing entranced me.

'You still doing film stuff?' he asked, and I remembered the night we celebrated my first big break in the movie industry with beers and laughter, me talking about changing the world, him asking me to be my escort to the Oscars.

'Yep, still pretending to be a Hollywood bigwig, and planning the socialist overthrow of the system.'

He laughed. 'You haven't changed,' he said, and poked me gently.

But I have, I wanted to say: *I am trying to be a different woman now. I have become less fearful than I was with you. I am no longer filled with self-hatred and doubt. I have no need to sabotage situations to protect my fragile and damaged ego. I am more able to express my feelings. I am learning that it is OK to love, even if it means losing someone. I am more able to face and deal with rejection, even when it hurts. I am seeing how it is better to risk pain than have a cold heart and be lonely. I am beginning to understand that real happiness can come from sharing pleasure, love and intimacy with another, not just from multiple orgasms.*

I felt an impulse to reach out to him – touch his face – tell him how much I regretted the way things ended between us, but no words came to me.

'What has it been? Seven years?' I asked, knowing exactly how long it was.

'Something like that. You look great,' he added.

I saw his eyes run over my body as if he was visualising me naked and I felt very self-conscious. I was haggard from the long flight and knew I looked rough. He looked me up and down and I remembered him kissing me from head to toe, following the contours of my body with his fingers, the way he loved my breasts and would spend an age caressing them, his cock rising as his hands stroked my nipples. He used to tell me I was beautiful, but I never believed him; I wondered if he still found me pretty.

'You look great too,' I responded, and meant it.

He had filled out a lot since I last saw him, but it suited him in that burly, manly way that tall men can sexily get away with. I remembered kissing his beer belly, laughing at the way it wobbled as I blew raspberries on it. I recalled grabbing hold of his love handles and pulling him close as he slid his cock inside me. Once I wrote his name in kisses on his back and I hoped he still knew how much I cared about him.

My ride from the airport arrived and cut the reminiscing short. We quickly exchanged numbers and swore we'd keep in touch, but I knew that we wouldn't speak again. It seemed right somehow to have closure this way – the coincidence of bumping into each other and finally ending that particular chapter in our lives.

As I walked away from him, I felt a distant thud in my heart. Not because I wanted him back in my life, and not out of regret for something I did in the past, but because I realised that he represented what it is that I now miss – loving someone, and being loved in return. Seeing him has made me see that I think I would like to share my life with someone special again.

The taxi headed towards Harry's apartment and as the city streets flashed by, I became aware of my loneliness and sadness about how things have turned out with Blog Boy. I still felt hopeful for the future: if I could meet my past in such a chance event, then surely it would just be a matter of time before serendipity crossed my path again offering my future.

I watched the sun begin to rise over the skyscrapers, and felt like this was a metaphor for my life: it was a new dawn and I was ready to feel the warmth of the sun, even if it burnt my eyes.

Thursday 3rd November

It's so nice to be back in New York, seeing Harry and my other old friends again. I do love to potter around this city. I've always felt an affinity to it, more so than London. Maybe it's because I visited here a lot as a child, with my parents, or perhaps it's because in this city I get chatted up constantly and I barely need to make an effort.

I just got approached by a guy on a subway train when I was making my way to see some friends on the Upper East Side – if that's not keen, I don't know what is. He was very cute – a little dishevelled, a slightly mischievous look, and when he walked up to me to ask if the diverted train I was stepping onto was heading uptown, I felt a little throb between my legs.

Neither of us could figure out the train route so we ended up chatting for over an hour as the subway went all round the houses. It was nice to have the company, especially when it was accompanied by his sexy smile.

He seemed quite sweet and eager, asking for my number and then texting me before I'd even got out of the subway station. That's all good. We've arranged to meet for a drink in a couple of days and I'm quite looking forward to it.

Harry, however, thinks I am insane to have a date with a complete stranger:

'What if he is a nutter?' he argued, as I staggered into his apartment slightly pissed tonight.

If he only knew what I'd done with all the other strangers I have met this year, he would have a fit.

Diary of a Sex Fiend

Saturday 5th November

We both laughed out loud and I noticed our knees touching.

Good sign, I thought, as I took another sip of my beer, perhaps a snog is on the cards.

It had all been going well with the guy from the train. After a few days' worth of flirtatious phone calls we were now relaxing in a bar which proudly displayed a flag proclaiming:

We, the people, say NO to the Bush agenda.

'Fantastic,' I said to myself, as I bought another round of beers, 'and impressive – obviously this guy is on the same page as me.'

Tipping the bartender, I noticed a sign above the bar and grinned as I read the caption:

George W. Bush couldn't run a laundromat; someone else for President.

Three thousand miles away from London and I felt at home. These were clearly my people.

It wasn't a far stretch to assume that this guy would be similarly like-minded; after all, he brought me to the place and if, like me, he's openly a leftie in his politics, then it was likely he would be open-minded about other things too.

I mentally checked off a wish-list of things to discuss in order to find out exactly how liberated he was:

1) casual sex
2) blow-job techniques
3) sex in public
4) spanking
5) threesomes

Then I realised that my list was entirely sex based and that I should probably try to impress him with my dazzling wit, knowledge about the movie industry and political know-how, instead of letting on that I am a sex fiend.

That could come later.

So I walked back to where he sat, expecting – and hoping – to have a stimulating discussion about the current political status of America and the potential fall-out for the Republican Party from Hurricane Katrina.

I was rather surprised when instead, he began to tell me about his prayer group meetings, how religious observance is the answer to life's ills and how the problems we see today are a result of sex before marriage.

I could have hit myself. I knew that he was from the South – and a farm boy at that – but I had tried not jump to conclusions. It seemed, sadly, that he was just a stereotypical Southern redneck God-botherer. Goddamit.

Here I was, a girl with a one-track mind, deep in discussion with someone who, if he knew the level of sordidness going on in my head, would have had to create a special prayer to God, just for me, in order to save me from all the sins I have performed (and hopefully am yet to perform) and save my soul.

I realised that if there was any spiritual searching to be done that night it didn't involve his lips and tongue finding the answers somewhere on my body.

Shit. How can I get out of this date? I racked my brain. I didn't want to offend him. He had invited me, after all, and it would be rude to leave abruptly. But I had to get away and other than mortally offending him by blaspheming and trashing his beliefs, my only get-out was to talk about sex. I reckoned that if I was graphic enough, I might embarrass him, and thus he would call an end to the night. Hallelujah.

So I elaborated on my theory, as proven by my ex, Rupert, that if more men teased women and refused them access to their cocks, it would drive women so crazy that they would eventually beg to be fucked, resulting in more orgasms and sex all round.

Then I argued that women are not as hung up about penis size as men are, and that if more guys relaxed about it, they would understand that when a woman is turned on, they don't give a fuck what is stuck in there, as long as 'you stick it in me now, oh God, fuck me, please fuck me'.

However, I was respectful and decent and didn't mention anal sex once. I am a lady, after all.

And oh heavenly joy, it seemed to work: he started shifting in his seat and blushing and looking rather uncomfortable. He looked at his watch and started making his excuses, and then we both agreed to call it a night and I made my way home – alone.

It did occur to me when I lay in bed, that at the same time, back in his own bedroom, he might have been praying for me and hoping that he'd saved me.

I prefer to think he finished off the evening more productively though, and that his hands were otherwise occupied.

Mine certainly were.

Monday 7th November

I love New York. I love the people. I love the atmosphere. I love their fantastic whisky sours that taste like nothing else on earth. And I love that I can get fingered by a complete stranger in a club and no one thinks anything of it.

As luck would have it, Tim just arrived in New York, on some last-minute business for his IT company. He called me just after he landed at the airport and excitedly demanded we meet up.

'Abby, I've read about the *perfect* place for us to go for a drink. It's a club where people go to hook up.'

'Another swingers, spa?' I asked.

'No, a club. Kind of swinger-lite,' he replied. 'The girls get it on and the men just stand back and watch. I read a review about it in *Time Out*.'

'What about your girl. I thought you weren't going to dabble without her?'

Tim paused. 'It didn't work out. She got back with her ex a couple of weeks ago. Actually, Abby, I could really do with going out right now. Why don't we just go and check it out, have some drinks and chat to some people? I need to have some fun.'

It did indeed sound fun. Let's face it, I haven't had much of that myself recently, either. So it didn't take a lot for Tim to talk me into it. A few hours later, clad in a black wrap dress, four-inch stilettos and no underwear – so I didn't break up the smooth lines of my tight dress, you see – I met up with him at the club.

The place itself was pretty standard: a long bar, some seats round the edge, a dance floor in the middle. Beautiful people in their twenties and thirties milled about smiling. It all seemed normal. Apart from the semi-naked women dancing on the podiums, that is.

Tim spotted them straight away and grinned at me. I pointed out one of them to him.

'She's fully shaved,' I teased, and Tim immediately groaned with desire as she bent over and we got a full view of her privates.

This was my kind of place indeed.

We gulped down a few drinks and got merry. The place began to get packed with people and Tim and I settled by the bar, body-watching.

'What do you think of her?' I asked, as a slim blonde woman walked past us.

'Not as much as I think of *her*,' Tim replied, pointing at a voluptuous Latina woman standing near us at the bar.

'Ooh, lovely. Just your type with her fab arse. Don't let me stand in your way,' I said, moving over to the other side of him so he would have full access and start chatting her up.

'Cheers, my dear,' Tim said, winking, and he set to work flirting with her.

I stood with my back to the bar and looked around once more. All of a sudden everyone seemed a bit less dressed – many of the girls had removed their tops. It occurred to me that perhaps I might get to see more action than just the stripping, and moments later, my suspicions were confirmed.

A few girls began to kiss each other and, right in front of me, two girls began to grope in full view of everyone. I watched as one of them slid her fingers under the other one's skirt, making her gasp in delight as she reached between her legs and kissed her in a frenzy. They snogged, groped and fondled each other and all the while their male partners stood by, rubbing up behind them.

God, it was hot. I was so jealous. What I would have given to have a partner at that moment, his cock rubbing up behind me as I groped some sexy girl's tits.

I was watching so intently that I didn't notice a man standing close to me until he whispered in my ear.

'Hot, isn't it?' he asked and smiled at me softly.

Shocked, I took a step back for a moment and looked him up and down.

He was *cute*. Lovely green eyes and a dazzling smile. My mind raced with possibilities.

'Yes,' I replied. 'Very sexy,' I smiled at him shyly.

'Lovely English accent you've got,' he said and grinned again. God, that smile was infectious. I felt myself melting in front of him.

We started chatting.

I'm not sure how long it was before I felt his hand softly caressing my arse, but however it got there, I didn't want him to stop: it felt delightful. And with all the alcohol, naughty goings-on around me and the slickness starting up between my legs, I wanted him to go further too.

'You're not wearing any underwear,' he remarked and looked at me slyly as his hand slowly lifted my dress and I felt the heat of his palm against my cool skin.

'Mmm,' I replied, not caring that my bare arse was on display.

He shifted behind me so his back was against the bar, keeping his hand on my backside the whole time. I felt him press his body against me and then I felt the delicious familiarity of an erect dick pushed up against my arse cheek. I moved against him, both his hands gripping my bum now.

'God, you have a great ass,' he exclaimed in his New York drawl. 'Fucking sexy. It's so damn firm.' He gave it a tight squeeze and I felt myself throb: I was so turned on already.

As if he read my mind, he then slowly slid his right hand between my legs.

'Fuck, you're wet!' he remarked. 'Jesus!' And with that he pushed two fingers inside me.

I suddenly became aware of what was going on: I was (yet again) getting felt up in a club, surrounded by people. How much of a sex fiend have I become? As he softly twisted his fingers inside me, I looked around at everyone, embarrassed.

But all around me were people in various states of undress, breasts on display, fingers in crotches. Well, that was a change – I wasn't the only one for once. Nobody was watching me. Tim was too busy snogging the Latina girl to notice my hot hand action.

Fuck it, I thought, I need some release. And so I let go, I relaxed into the hand job I was receiving; a few moments later I was dripping onto his hand, climaxing hard.

When I had finished shaking, he kissed me softly on the neck.

'That was wonderful,' he said. 'You're a sexy woman, do you know that?'

I turned to face him. 'Thanks,' I replied. 'You've made my holiday very special.'

We stood watching the floorshow together until Tim's jetlag got too much and he dragged me off before the dawn broke.

I kissed the cute New Yorker goodbye on my way out and he thrust his card in my hand, telling me to call him if I wanted some more fun sometime.

I clutched his card carefully. I may just need it.

Tuesday 8th November

Met up with Harry for brunch in his local diner today, a bit worse for wear. I didn't see him when I got in last night, and he was up before me this morning. He laughed when he saw me totter in – the evidence of my late night showing clearly on my exhausted face.

He wanted to know where I'd been and teased me mercilessly until I finally caved in and told him how I got lucky last night.

Congratulating me, Harry ordered me some strong coffee and we settled down to a hearty meal of cheese blintzes and waffles.

Over my third cup of coffee, Harry probed me a little more.

'So do you like this guy from last night, then?'

I nodded. 'Sure, he's a nice guy; we had fun.'

'Just a *shag*, then,' Harry said, impersonating my English accent.

'You got it,' I replied laughing and took another gulp of coffee.

Harry pondered for a moment. 'So,' he said, 'whatever happened to that blogger you met; the one you let feel you up in the middle of Oxford Street?'

I practically spat out my coffee. I had forgotten I'd told Harry about Blog Boy. How I had just met him when I came to New York in January. How I had been so excited about getting back to London for our third date. How much I had liked him. How I had hoped for something to develop.

I suddenly felt tears well up in my eyes and I was lost for words.

Harry looked at me and took my hand, 'Oh, Abby, I'm sorry. Are you OK?'

I nodded through the tears and fidgeted with my coffee cup, trying to find the words.

'It's just … it's stupid, that's all.'

'What is?'

'Me. I am a twat.'

'Why?'

'Because. Because I said I would never be one of those women who mix up sex and love and I think I have become one.'

Harry looked confused. 'I don't understand, Abby. What happened?'

I sighed deeply. 'I don't know. I don't get it. When I got back from New York, we seemed to be getting along fine. Then he said he just wanted to be friends.'

'Friends?' Harry said, suspiciously. 'After hitching your skirt up and everything?'

'Yup; he was going travelling and didn't want to get involved,' I explained. 'So we became friends, hung out and stuff; it all seemed fine. And you know, I continued dating and having fun; *lots* of fun. But then a few months ago, we slept together.'

'Ah,' Harry said, 'I see,' and he nodded in understanding.

'Three times,' I added.

'Right,' he replied.

'Which,' I continued, 'I know means nothing, but after getting to know him over six months, it didn't feel like they were just one-night stands – you know?'

Harry nodded.

'So then he went away and we didn't speak. But now he has been emailing me again and we're going to meet when I get back to London. And I guess I'm hoping that we might get into something. I'd like to – I think.'

'So tell him what you want,' Harry said. 'Just tell him.'

I shook my head. 'I can't. I just can't.'

'Do you mean to tell me, you can have sex with a complete stranger, but you are unable to tell Blog Boy what's on your mind?'

'Yes, stupid, I know.'

'Abby, I know you. You are an honest and upfront woman – in fact you're the most straightforward person I know. Why can't you tell him what's on your mind?'

I shrugged. 'Harry, it's not that simple; we're not "in" something – how can I say I think I want more from him? And do I really – I mean, I am having a good time right now, so do I really want to be with him?'

'The question you need to be asking yourself is how long can you *not* say anything? It's obvious to me that you want more – and if you're not getting it, something has to change,' Harry said firmly.

I stayed silent. Harry continued.

'If you want to give things a try with him, then do. When he gets back from his vacation, talk to him and see what happens. And if you don't, then at least try to make sure you have some more good shags lined up.'

I looked up and saw Harry grinning at me. I smiled back. He was right. Especially about the shags.

Wednesday 9th November

I watched the contortionist wrap his legs behind his ears and rest his chin on top of his crotch. One thought immediately came to mind, and I whispered it to the person next to me.

It was such an instant, instinctive thought that its implications didn't dawn on me until I'd already made my little witticism. It was the mental image of the contortionist sucking his own cock.

And what I had whispered was, 'I bet he can auto-fellate.'

And the person I had leaned over and said this to happened to be my mother – also on holiday in New York.

As the realisation of what I had just done began to hit me, the dreaded – most feared – words came out of my mother's mouth. I watched her lips purse together, and in slow-motion movie-style, say, 'What's auto-fellate?'

I sat there silently for a moment and thought of my options.

★ Lying is not something I am good at, and I tend to avoid because it is inevitably followed by sleepless nights in which I rack my conscience.

★ Pleading ignorance wouldn't work either: my mother knows me too well. The only reason I would use a technical term for something is if I actually knew what it meant.

★ And the truth? Well, I've been in a similar situation with her before and it didn't turn out all bad. Surely the best choice.

So I said, softly, to my own mother, 'It's when a guy has the ability to suck his own cock.'

My mother looked at me, and blushed. 'What?' she said, 'I didn't hear you properly. Tell me again.'

I groaned inwardly. If there was a God now would be a good time to strike me down. 'Auto-fellatio is when a guy has the ability to suck his own cock,' I repeated, adding, 'supposedly two men out of every hundred are able to do it,' as if that statistic would somehow make it all alright.

My mother looked at me, baffled. I thought it might help if I said no more, so instead I motioned with my head in a downward bobbing movement to try to show what I was talking about.

It was probably the worst rendition of self-induced oral sex in the history of mime, but I didn't care to show off my cock-sucking skills to my mother. She's seen enough – she doesn't need to know what my own personalised blow-job technique looks like.

Thankfully, my mother stopped blushing and instead slowly nodded in recognition of my explanation/badly performed charade. But, as if possessed by some kind of truth demon, I couldn't stop myself blurting out, 'He is definitely able, look at him!', and pointing to the contortionist as he crab-walked around the Sixth Avenue Manhattan theatre with his head still sitting on his crotch.

My mother turned to look, and I tried to erase from my brain the fact that my mother was now mentally picturing the acrobat merrily slurping away on his own penis.

This was all becoming far too psychologically complex for me, and when my dad – who was seated the other side of me – chipped in and said 'What are you two talking about?', I felt like I was going to die of embarrassment and self-induced neurosis.

I waited, with a heavy knot in my stomach, for my mother to respond.

'Oh, we were just saying how athletic and fit the performer must be,' she explained to my dad. 'He is so flexible, isn't he?'

She turned to look back at the contortionist and we all continued watching his amazing performance. I thought that was the end of it, and hoped I could put this episode behind me.

A moment later though, my mother leaned over to me. 'I think you're right,' she said and winked at me, before turning back to watch the rest of the show.

I sat, mortified, and waited for it to end; the sooner I could escape back to Harry's apartment and recount the story to him in all its awkwardness, the better.

Thursday 10th November

By coincidence, I notice that David Lynch's awesome film *Mulholland Drive* is screening on American television tonight. Coincidence because I first watched that film with my parents, and for horror, inappropriateness and sheer, mind-numbing embarrassment, that occasion was more than the equal of last night's circus outing.

A few years ago, I had some preview tickets for the film and decided to take my mum and dad, since they – like me – are huge Lynch fans.

In the first hour I developed a little crush on Rita (the actress Laura Harring). She was beautiful: a sultry brunette with a seductive voice, oozing femininity. She had the most fantastic body: curvaceous, womanly, and with wonderful, glorious breasts that I found mesmerising. If there was any woman on earth that I would like to shag, it is her. Suffice to say I had been feeling a warm throb between my legs for a while.

So when Rita entered the bedroom wearing only a towel

and Betty (Naomi Watts) suggested that she join her in the bed too, I was quite excited: some nice nudity – great.

I wasn't wrong. Rita immediately disposed of the towel, revealing her voluptuous torso silhouetted in the half-light, and then slid into bed with Betty.

I sat there thinking – no, *wishing* – that they would get it on. And they do. It was fucking hot: two women exploring each other hungrily, passionately. It was photographed so sensually that it was difficult for me not to attempt to rub one out there and then. I shifted and squirmed in my seat, feeling the heat.

Then I remembered. I was sitting next to my parents. They were watching the same sex scene. There I was, horny as hell, wanting a fiddle and my parents were next to me.

That's when it struck me: the one thing you do not want to think about when you think about your parents. That is, that they might be horny too.

Now, I don't think I'm jumping to conclusions here. I know I was, like the majority of the audience in the cinema that night, blown away by the erotic content. It wasn't such a huge leap to imagine (yuck) that my parents might find it a turn-on too.

I didn't want to think about it any further, but it was at least a great passion-killer, and I was able to watch the rest of the scene as long as I stared straight ahead and ignored any movement on either side of me.

I thought I was doing OK too. The movie continued in its dream-like non-linear narrative and I became immersed in the way I was pulled into the story and then had tricks played with my expectations. I began to relax a little and enjoy it all once more. That was until the masturbation scene.

David Lynch should have provided a disclaimer prior to the movie, to prepare me for the embarrassment of having to watch a woman frig herself into oblivion on screen in front of my parents. It was awful.

But as cringingly uncomfortable as I felt, I was compelled to watch the whole thing. I thought it was shot beautifully – almost worth watching just to see how realistically the portrayal of female masturbation can be filmed. Ninety per cent of the porn I've seen makes it look completely fake and unsexy.

The character Diane (Naomi Watts again) is trying to pleasure herself after being dumped by Camilla (Laura Harring again). We see and hear her as she gets near to her climax, her vision keeps blurring, her face sets in a tight grimace at her frustration at not being able to orgasm. She rubs harder and harder and eventually is rewarded with her release – a literal analogy of her accepting the break-up. After she comes, her vision is clear again: beautiful.

I watched it and thought, Yeah, I can relate to that. So fucking frustrating when it can take that long to come, and horrible when it's a result of being so emotionally distraught, and I turned around half expecting the rest of the audience to be nodding their heads in appreciation too, and then I remembered once more that I was surrounded by my parents.

Who have just been watching a young woman pretending to masturbate on screen. I think I physically shuddered, I was so uncomfortable. But there was nothing else to be done – if I dodged out of the auditorium how the hell would I explain myself? No, I had to stick it out to the end.

I was rewarded with grateful thanks from my parents, who said 'It was the best movie exploring the unconscious mind they had ever seen' and that 'Lynch has a wonderful imagination.'

Thank fuck for that. Long-term Parental Cringe Avoidance Strategy not needed: my parents were unharmed and my reputation as a well-brought-up daughter was maintained – even though they never discussed the movie ever again and I am still too embarrassed to mention it to them.

But there were some bonuses that came from seeing this film. I took my boyfriend Rupert to watch it soon after and told him to squeeze my hand any and every time he felt like he was getting an erection from anything on screen.

He squeezed it almost continuously for 90 minutes. So as soon as the movie finished, I pushed him into a cab and then fucked his brains out when we got home.

A happy ending if there ever was one.

Friday 11th November

Harry and I hugged each other tightly.

'I'm going to miss you,' I said.

He nodded at me, the tears in his eyes reflecting the ones welling up in my own, 'Me too.'

I looked at him – my oldest friend in the world – and felt my heart ache. Why did he have to be three thousand miles away? And would I ever feel the way I feel about him about any other man? Would I be able to love someone as deeply?

I felt an impulse to tell him I loved him and that he had a place in my heart that no one else has ever reached, that leaving him was almost too painful to bear.

As if he read my mind, Harry held my hand. 'You don't need to say it,' he said, 'I know.'

I smiled at him through my tears and we hugged once more.

'Now go, Abby. I'll see you soon.' He grinned at me.

I nodded and picked up my bags. As I got into the cab, Harry called out to me once more.

'Good luck,' he said and we both knew what he was talking about.

Saturday 12th November

'You're my favourite lady,' the stewardess on the plane back to London breathed, as she leant in towards me.

'Really?' I said, catching a whiff of her delicate perfume and getting another glimpse of her ample cleavage plunging in the neckline of her tight, white shirt.

'Yes, you're the nicest one here – so polite. I've been calling you "nice lady" to the others.'

I smiled shyly, and tried not to stare at her large, perfectly round bosoms, as they were thrust in my face.

'Well, um, thanks. You've really been so helpful.'

'Oh, it's my pleasure,' she said as she handed me my drink, 'it's always lovely to have someone like you on board.'

Her fingers lingered on mine for a second as I took the small plastic cup from her. It was a tiny gesture – and very ambiguous – and if we had been in any other environment it might have been far more meaningful.

'Is that OK?' she asked, gesturing towards my drink, 'I opened a new bottle for you, but I wasn't sure how much soda to add.'

She waited for me to sip it. I suddenly felt very self-conscious. There were 200 other people on board the aircraft and she was waiting on me as if it were just the two of us. My hand shook a little and I wondered whether there was turbulence. There was certainly fluttering going on between my legs.

'I can get you another one if you don't like it,' she said, still waiting for my response.

I quickly tasted the drink. It was perfect – the best ratio of Scotch to soda water that a top bartender could have mixed – but that wasn't the point. She needed my appreciation.

'My God, that is delicious,' I remarked, as I took another gulp, 'fantastic. Thank you so much, it's lovely. I really appreciate your doing this for me.'

She breathed a sigh of relief, and I tried not to look at her heaving bosom stretching the thin material of her uniform. I also tried not to look at her erect nipples poking through.

'I'm glad you like it. If you want another one – or anything else – you just call for me; my name is Kelly.' She beamed at me.

'Thank you, I will,' I responded, and noticed how pretty her green eyes were and how soft and kissable her mouth looked. 'You've been very kind.'

'And you're very nice,' she replied, 'just call if you need me.' She smiled again and wandered off to the galley.

I sat there, drink in hand and watched her elegant legs walk away from me, her fine arse beautifully sculpted in her tight skirt. I tried to collect my thoughts. Was she flirting with me? Did her gestures mean anything? How long would I be able to wait before popping to the loo to do something with the mental image that whole train of thought had given me?

It couldn't wait. A few minutes later I got up from my seat and made my way to the toilet. Damn, a queue. I waited in line, and noticing my own erect nipples through my top, willing them into submission. It didn't work.

'It's my nice lady again.'

I turned to find her behind me. I smiled, and she squeezed past me to make her way down the aisle.

Though the space was narrow, there was room for two people to pass, so I was slightly surprised – but not at all disappointed – when she pushed right up against me as she moved by.

Smelling her sweet perfume, and feeling her soft breasts squeezed against mine, was almost too much for me. I wanted to grab her bum then and there, pull her close, kiss her deeply and run my fingers across her ample bosom.

But the moment was all too brief. She was gone and I was left dripping wet with a need to do something about it – quick.

As soon as the toilet was free, I rushed in to sort myself out, picturing her sitting on my lap with her skirt hitched to her waist and her breasts in my mouth.

Moments later I was climaxing. It was fast, furious and lots of fun – much like my trip to New York.

Monday 14th November

I feel refreshed once more. New York has lifted me; I feel ready for new challenges in my life. And that includes Blog Boy. If our shagging did mean more than just sex to him, then maybe I should give things a try, now that we're both back in town.

But I don't think I should sleep with him unless I know he does feel the same way. It would just confuse things.

It's going to be hard for me to achieve though. I am gagging for another shag right now.

Saturday 19th November

Ironic that after meeting the Southern farm boy in New York, I then come back to London and spend all of last night once again in the company of a group of religious fanatics.

That's right, me. Girl with a one-track mind – the sex-obsessed atheist, in a party full of God-botherers. It was like torture, and not the enjoyable mild BDSM-type either.

It wasn't my usual Saturday night's entertainment, it has to be said. I went to my elderly relative's party with an open mind, figuring that if my great-uncle wanted to celebrate with a few hymns and stuff, I would understand.

I wasn't prepared for a full-on Billy Graham revival, complete with prayers, speeches by religious leaders and choral singing to the accompaniment of a band:

'*Jesus ... must be obeyed;*
There is ... no other way.'

Christ. What the hell had I got myself into?

There I was, sitting in a room filled with people praising the Lord every other minute and I felt like a traitor, an outsider. Their belief system and mine were diametrically opposed.

As they sang God's praises and clapped their hands in glee, I knew I was out of place. I had nothing in common with these folk – apart from the fact that we were sipping the same wine – how the hell could I have a decent conversation with anyone, when I believed them all to be completely deluded?

It struck me that if the people in there knew just one per cent of what occupied my mind at any given minute, they would have been horrified:

Diary of a Sex Fiend

★ A sex fiend?

★ A girl who loves cock?

★ A multi-orgasmic, permanently aroused sex obsessive?

A preacher would have a field day with me – they could cast me out as a Sinner, pray for Divine Intervention, or make me beg for my Redemption – hours of fun.

Bored out of my mind and affronted by all the religious propaganda, I suddenly got this impulse to stand up and do something totally improper, sordid and lewd, confronting my great-uncle and showing him that I was no longer the polite, innocent girl he thought me to be.

Reckon I need guidance? I'll get on my knees and worship in public, if God is a cock and answering my prayers means corresponding directly with my mouth.

Think sex is evil? Well then, how about I dress head to foot in a black rubber cat-suit, complemented by knee-high stiletto-heeled boots and topped off with a studded collar round my neck to show you just how corrupt I now am?

Believe that I need to repent? I've learned I can be a bad girl, so give me a six-foot whip in my hand, some adoring worshipper at my feet and the chance to dish out some punishment to his willing backside (and, yeah, I'd graciously allow him to become my tongue slave after he had begged for mercy as part of his redemption, too), and then maybe I could recognise the error of my ways.

The daydream went no further than this though, sadly. I didn't even say the word 'fuck', I was so well behaved.

I think a few of the congregation might have had heart attacks, had I gone through with the fantasy – even though those would just be the ones who were secret hard-core S&M porn fans.

Hopefully that wouldn't include my great-uncle. Rubber wouldn't suit him.

Friday 25th November

I ended up sleeping with Blog Boy again last night. I tried not to, I really did. I wanted to see how he felt about everything before I shagged him, but I couldn't help myself. It's been months since we last saw each other and now we're both back in town, it just seemed natural for us to end up in bed again at the end of the evening.

So after much food and wine we ended up at his place, falling into each other's arms and having pretty passionate sex. It was lovely. We seem to fit together so well, we match each other, both in drive and in pleasure.

But today, when Blog Boy had to go to work, he seemed to cold shoulder me once again. Perhaps I am being neurotic, but it sort of felt like I was some kind of regretted one-night stand. Maybe that is what I am to him – I don't know. I'm so confused now.

What I do know is that no matter how hard I have tried, I cannot help but have feelings for him – even when I haven't seen him for so long. They've just got more intense in the meantime. Every time I have seen him, every time I have slept with him, it's just reinforced how I feel.

So when his arms were wrapped around me as we dozed off together, I felt happy and wanted, and I knew that – with him – it wasn't, nor has it ever been, just about the sex for me.

As for him, I don't know. I am worried that if I were to tell him how I really feel, he might stop seeing me. And though I know it's stupid, that it's not good for me, at least having a little of something with him is better than nothing at all.

Even though it is beginning to eat me up inside.

The Girl's Guide to Fuck-Buddies

What to do if you end up having sex with a friend:

1 Whether or not sex is involved, a friendship must be built on trust, honesty and openness, and these things take priority over any sexual desires. If this is not the case, it cannot survive sex entering the equation.

2 You cannot treat your mate like you would a fuck-buddy. The latter will not be offended if you are out of contact for some time or decline to meet up, but a friend may feel rejected if you do not make arrangements to see them in a non-sexual context too.

3 Wants and needs are fluid things and should be constantly reassessed and talked about. Whereas two months ago, one person may have just wanted a drunken grope with their mate, now they may have feelings for the other person. If this is not discussed, the boundaries of the friendship will be threatened and the relationship risks failing.

4 Understand that the sex may be more intimate than fuck-buddy sex. The very nature of friendship means that the experience will involve more than basic physical sexual expression. Beware that this doesn't necessarily mean anything more than what it in fact is: emotional closeness expressed through sexual physicality.

5 Do not have sex with your friends if:
a) You have romantic feelings for them. It will only mess with your head and your heart, and, inevitably, your friendship too.

b) You find it hard to have emotionally disconnected sex. Shagging someone you don't care about can be hard in itself when it comes to merely forming a physical connection; shagging someone you do care about, even if it's only platonically, can make the experience painful at best, and emotionally damaging at worst.

c) You really want to be in a relationship with *someone*, and even though you may not harbour romantic feelings for your friend, you know that having sex with them and experiencing that closeness will remind you of what you are missing, and what you really want. Bound to result in regret and an unpleasant aftertaste.

12

December

Thursday 1st December

It's funny. After Steven, I wanted to avoid getting involved with anyone. All I wanted was to have a good time without the hassle of a relationship, but meeting Blog Boy threw me. Here was a bloke that I liked, that I could actually imagine being with – a man I didn't just want to fuck.

So why has sleeping with him again left my head in such a mess? Why has it made me so confused? Surely I should know where things are at between us now – it's been long enough.

But I don't know, and it's no good. I have to tell him how I feel and find out if he feels the same. If he doesn't, I don't want to sleep with him again. Even though he makes my pants wet, just being a fuck-buddy isn't enough for me – I want and deserve more.

So maybe I need to wait until I next see him, before I have sex again – with anyone – because I need to know if he's worth being the only man in my life. It is going to be hard for me – I wouldn't mind another shag and turning away temptation will be a challenge, but I think I need to give it a try – for now, anyway.

Diary of a Sex Fiend

Sunday 4th December

Sometimes all it takes is a look.

I felt him staring at me even before I looked up to meet his eyes. I was aware of his piercing gaze, and knew that out of all the people at my great-aunt's birthday party, he was looking solely at me.

Over the last few months I have learned that occasionally instant chemistry occurs. I don't think it has anything to do with fancying, or flirtation, or even curiosity. It is just synchronisation on a purely physical and carnal level: across a room two people can share a glance and immediately know that they want to fuck each other's brains out.

When I saw the way this guy looked at me today, I knew. The hunger, the way he held my gaze without looking away, not smiling, yet with desire clearly shining – I could feel it burning into me even though he was standing some distance away. The sexual tension hung in the air like an invisible mist, his body screaming out loudly to me over the chatter of the party. He watched my face and waited for my response.

I was trying to think with some clarity, rather than listen to the pulse beating between my legs as I watched him watching me. I had no misconceptions here. There would be no getting to know each other, no friendly chat over drinks, no knowing of names. This would be him pushing me against the wall of the toilet cubicle, pulling up my dress, tugging my thong to one side and ramming his cock into me. We would be two strangers clawing at each other, fucking with fury, dripping with sweat, and then moments later, we would dress and rejoin the party. We'd carry on without even missing a beat.

As I looked at him, I knew all of this lay ahead. I've been here before and I know a zipless fuck when I see one.

My pussy throbbed. I knew he would be getting hard too: I saw him adjust himself as he continued watching me and I wondered why I was attracted to him.

Here was a man, 20 years my senior, rotund, short, and with all the typical mannerisms of an East End wheeler-dealer geezer. It certainly wasn't his appearance, or the twang of his cockney voice, which filled me with desire. Nor was it his age. Unless it was David Lynch talking to me all night, older men do not interest me. No, it was the way he looked at me – the assured steadiness of his gaze – it let me know that he wanted to fuck me, and that, pure and simple, is what made me so aroused right there in the middle of my great-aunt's do.

I debated what to do. It was my choice after all. I knew that if I kept eye contact and walked into the toilet, he would have followed me. It excited me that sex was so clearly within my grasp, that I could enter the loo and then be pummelled by him shortly afterwards. I imagined what it would be like having his breath on my neck and his cock between my legs. I could almost feel the orgasm I would have had, welling up inside me ready to burst. I wanted him badly.

I stared at him, and thought for a moment. As much as I yearned to fuck him, I knew I couldn't. I knew I shouldn't. I knew it wasn't right for me to do it. I was at the party as a carer for my great-aunt, and going off to the bathroom for a quick fuck would mean leaving her to fend for herself. I couldn't do that to her, as much as I wanted a shag.

I also thought about Blog Boy. If he is as important to me as I'd like him to be, surely I shouldn't be shagging other blokes too? Maybe, I thought, if I don't have sex with anyone else, then things will fall into place with him. It's worth a try.

So I broke my stare with the older man. He kept glancing over at me for the rest of the evening, but I chose to look away. The temptation to act was far too strong.

Unfortunately, when it comes to my desire, I have discovered that I am more of a looter who impatiently breaks all the glass to steal what's on display, rather than a patient, well-behaved shopper queuing at a checkout. I have become a great pursuer of the 'try before you buy' type deals on offer.

However, if today is anything to go by, I guess I'm learning how to slowly window-shop instead, or at least, now I'll remove the window carefully before grabbing the goods – a definite improvement in my eyes – even though it meant I lost out on a hearty rogering. I still managed to retain my will power, which for me, is quite an achievement.

Friday 9th December

Again, I've managed to turn down another shag. I elected to send a cute guy home alone this evening – and I am glad I did.

Kathy's friend Brian and I had a lovely meal, followed by some interesting conversation, helped along by many rounds of drinks. While we chatted I became aware of his body language. It's something I have been paying a lot of attention to during my explorations this year. I have discovered that it's a huge advantage to be fluent in the physical manifestations of people's unconscious desires. Knowing what someone's intentions might be, before they've expressed them verbally, has kept me one step ahead in the shagging field.

It seemed clear to me that Brian fancied me, but I didn't want to get involved:

1) He was much younger than me. Previous experience has shown me that although younger men may have good stamina in the sack, they rarely know how to deal with an older woman on an emotional level. Still developing their sense of self, they inevitably end up with their feelings hurt when faced with an independent woman who may only want a casual dalliance with them.

2) He admitted to me that he was very sexually inexperienced with women and that sex scared him. It wasn't the inexperience itself that put me off – I know that I could corrupt him in two minutes flat and that it would be hugely fun: 'Ooh look, someone I can mould into being a superb lover, and who'll be grateful for evermore; how delightful!'

That would stroke my ego, but the potential psychological damage I could cause in the meantime meant I should know better, and not touch him with a bargepole.

3) When he went to the bar to get more drinks, I saw someone who looked like Blog Boy and my heart leapt. It wasn't him, but my reaction to seeing him made me realise just how much I like Blog Boy – and want to be with him.

And again I thought to myself that if only I could control my desire and not give in to temptation and distractions, it might enable me to see if something more can develop between me and Blog Boy.

When Brian's hand grazed mine as he put down his pint glass, or when he touched my arm gently as he was making a point, I did not return the gestures. I did not laugh wildly at his jokes when I didn't mean it. I did not throw back my hair and twirl it nervously around my fingers.

And at the end of the night, when he leaned in to give me an open-mouthed kiss on the lips, I moved my face aside and let him find my cheek instead.

Because of Blog Boy, I am all too aware of the potential consequences of a one-night stand: someone may get their feelings hurt. So not wanting to be the cause of any pain on Brian's part, I said goodnight and made my way home.

As I got on the bus, I suddenly felt confused. I had sacrificed spending the night with someone because of a man who might not even want me – was I doing the right thing?

The bus drove off and I resigned myself to the thought that I had made the right choice regardless. I may have lost out on a potential shag, I may have felt lonely, but at least I could sleep with a clear conscience.

Although dreaming about Blog Boy didn't help me get much rest, it has to be said.

Monday 12th December

Dear Man on the Northern Line,

You may think I didn't notice how you scanned the carriage as you entered and made eye contact with me before sitting next to me.

Perhaps you observed how even though you were clearly a handsome chap, I only looked at you once, before pretending to fiddle with my iPod.

Maybe you knew that I would find someone like you very appealing. It is true that in your tall, blue-eyed, sexy mid-thirtyish way, I would consider you ripe and perfect for picking. You did, after all, remind me of Blog Boy and his looks. But suddenly I felt sad when I saw you, because you made me think of how much I like him.

So when you kept staring at my reflection in the window, and I turned to look away, I shall have you know that it was because I was thinking of him and trying to exercise my will power and self-control, and not because I wasn't interested in you.

Even when you half smiled at me and I felt compelled to grin back.

You see, you kept making it difficult for me with your ingenious, calculating, manly ways. When you spread your legs and ensured they rested against mine at all times, you must have known how hard it was for me not to place my hand on your thigh and squeeze it gently.

And when you slid your forearm alongside my own so that I could feel your warm skin against mine, it was surely obvious that I was fighting the urge to rest my fingers on yours and stroke them gently.

But when you then began to tense the muscles in your leg so that I could feel the movement up against my own thigh, it really was most out of order Don't you know that a woman like me is barely able to resist such a gesture?

The fact that it made me want to:

1) Slide my hand between your legs to feel your cock;
2) Raise my leg over yours and squeeze your thigh underneath mine;

3) Place your hand between my legs so you could feel my wetness.

And yet I still managed gently to move my own thigh away, while trying to maintain an air of decency. This shows that I do in fact have some resolution and even when faced with such a pussy-tease as you, I can exercise some self-control.

Or course it didn't help that:

1) I was thinking about what your cock would feel like inside me;
2) I was wondering whether you would be as good in bed as Blog Boy:
3) I was considering if you could be Boyfriend Potential Material.

But I managed to contain myself, even when faced with such a challenge.

I appreciate that you helped me strengthen my resolve, enabling me to delay acting out my desires until I got home, rather than attempting to get you into bed with me as I might have done a few months ago.

I am proud to say that I behaved like a lady, treating the situation with dignity and elegance. A truly classy performance all round, and one to be repeated – I hope.

(Except for that moment when I bent down slightly to give you a better view of my boobs, but let's not go into that now, even if it did give you some issues in the trouser department.)

Yours thankfully,

Abby

Wednesday 14th December

I just found an old email from Jake, a guy I was seeing three years ago. I couldn't read it without weeping – I'm such a girl sometimes. Or maybe it's just because I am feeling fragile right now, because yet again, I haven't heard from Blog Boy since we had sex and I can't bring myself to contact him right now.

Reading Jake's final email to me has made me wonder what he is up to nowadays, where he is at in his life. Whether he married the girlfriend he cheated on with me; if he finally has the kids that he so desired.

To this day, I am still racked with guilt about our brief 'affair'. It rests uneasily on my conscience – a reminder that someone will always be affected by the choices I make. I have to be responsible for my actions.

I've never been unfaithful to a guy. I'm probably old-fashioned like that. I am beginning to think that a monogamous relationship with a man is more of a sacred bond to me, rather than a bind – I want to be with one, special man and I think I am ready for it too.

I would also enjoy the excitement of having sex with another to add spice to our otherwise monogamous sex life – an occasional threesome with my partner could surely spice up the monotony of our twosome?

But this wasn't the arrangement that I, Jake and his girlfriend had. We snuck around behind her back, making quiet calls and sending brief texts to work out how and where we would next meet. Our dalliance was secretive, our relationship duplicitous.

I always thought that affairs were nasty things where you would find yourself stealing brief moments to shag senselessly.

Not so in this case. Perhaps the reason it affected us both so badly was that often we just met to talk, the physical contact limited to our eyes locking and our fingers touching. We had a connection, but it wasn't purely sexual.

Maybe this was what was so difficult about the whole episode. The Abby that Jake got to know was not the neurotic self-absorbed woman obsessed with sex, but the thoughtful idealist who wore her heart on her sleeve. He embraced that part – romanced it – and I felt completely at ease with him. I was able just to relax and be myself and he loved me all the more for it.

And, some months later, when we finally did make it into bed, he discovered my inner sex fiend too and made me feel like I was normal, rather than just needy. We made love with a passion and I felt connected to him on every level.

The guilt ate both of us up, though, and rightly so. Even though I regret doing something I can now see as morally wrong, I'm also glad I experienced being with him. Jake helped me be the woman I could be, one who is able to connect mentally with a lover and express her emotions. He showed me that there was a man out there who was so entranced by me that he would want to meet up with me just to talk, rather than fuck me. Jake made me see that I didn't have to battle between love and lust – that with the right person it, and I, will fall naturally into place.

So I look back on that situation with mixed emotions: feeling a longing for him and the closeness we had; feeling guilt about what we did; and feeling a pang in my heart because I miss having this connection with someone.

And now, when I think of Blog Boy, I wonder if this is what we have. Is our connection as deep? Or do his feelings for me lie closer to his cock than the depths of his heart?

Friday 16th December

'So, what do you think?'

I looked down at the package Tim had placed on the table and considered my response.

1) I could be honest. This would be the best result overall, but would mean he got the full wrath of my judgment.
2) I could lie. This would be immoral, but also ensure his feelings did not get hurt.
3) I could withhold my opinion. This would give him the opportunity to show off his purchase and receive the feedback he needed.

I chose the last. 'They're y-fronts,' I remarked nonchalantly, wondering if he would understand how much of a mistake I thought he had made with his pant-buying just by the tone of my voice.

'Yes,' he said excitedly, 'nice, aren't they?'

'Well, they're y-fronts,' I stated, thinking that perhaps if I just repeated myself that would eliminate any possibility of my being rude to him absentmindedly.

He picked up the packet of three white pants and handed them to me. 'Have a look. What do you reckon?'

I held the package in my hand and an image of him wearing y-fronts suddenly entered my head. Given that I normally like the thought of men in pants (especially if I have the chance to rip them off), it was not without some irony that I found myself trying to empty my mind of this particular thought. But even though I shagged him years ago, I really didn't want to think of Tim in that way again – especially not with y-fronts on.

I wondered how I could respond in the least offensive manner. Perhaps if I came up with a question, it would deflect attention away from my negative opinion and onto his enthusiasm instead.

'So, do you actually use the hole in the front, then?' I asked, prodding the pants through the plastic wrapping. 'Does it make for easy access?'

I looked up at him and suddenly took in the inappropriateness of my question. Another image of him in pants appeared in my head.

He stammered a little. 'Well, yes, of course. I mean—'

'Right,' I interrupted, fully aware that neither of us really wanted to be debating the merits of him being able to stick his cock through a front opening – of any sort. 'So they must be comfortable, I imagine?'

'Ooh yes, really comfy,' he said, sounding relieved I had moved the debate on. 'What size are you?'

'Me? I'm a medium. Why?'

'I reckon a man's small would fit you,' he said, adding 'and I have a pack of them at home.'

'But they're boys' pants!' I exclaimed, still trying to get the image of him modelling the y-fronts out of my head. 'I'm a girl!' *And no way would I wear anything like that.*

'You could look like Sarah Jessica Parker!' he said, excitedly.

'What?'

'She wore her boyfriend's y-fronts in *Sex and the City*. You could definitely get away with it like she did. They'd look great on you. I'll give you the spare pack I've got,' he went on.

Oh great. A bloke is reciting an episode of Sex and the City *to me. And he's not gay. And he thinks y-fronts look good on women too. Clearly he has no taste. Oh God, how do I get out of this without totally offending him?*

I weighed up my options for a moment and then came up with the best answer I could. Leaning over to him, I gently placed my hand on his and in my most seductive voice said, 'Why would a woman want to wear pants made for boys when there are the silkiest thongs, the laciest French knickers and the sheerest tie-string pants to choose from?'

He looked at me for a moment, thinking, and then said, somewhat triumphantly, 'Fair enough. But what about to sleep in, then, 'Eh?''

I smiled at him. 'My dear Tim, the joy of underwear is to take it *off* – preferably in front of someone else. There is never a need to wear pants to bed. At least, not in my bed.'

He laughed. 'OK, yeah, you're right, good point.'

'Save them for your next girlfriend,' I said, as he hurriedly put the packet of y-fronts away.

But we clearly still have some work to do if you're determined to stick with the y-fronts whilst dating.

Sunday 18th December

Earlier today:

'It'll take a while before it reformats,' Tom said, sitting back in the chair, as my laptop screen burst into action in front of him.

'Would you like some tea?' I asked, as he pushed himself away from the desk.

'No thanks, but I'd like something else,' he replied.

'What's that, then?' I asked, thinking perhaps he'd prefer a beer.

'I'd like for you to take off that t-shirt and show me your tits,' he responded.

I shouldn't have been shocked really; after all, the last time we were alone together he was spanking my arse hard as he fucked me from behind, but that was many months ago and things have changed for both of us since then – not least him getting back with his old girlfriend and me now really wanting to give things a go with Blog Boy.

'C'mon,' I said, trying to sound convincing, 'you know we're just friends now.'

'OK then, you can leave your bra on. I just want to see your lovely big bosoms outside that top.' He smiled at me wickedly and fixed his gaze on my nipples. I felt them begin to harden slightly and knew that he would be able to see their outline through my t-shirt.

'I'd really prefer not to,' I pleaded. 'How about a nice cuppa?'

'I'll just have to use my imagination then, Abby,' he said, and with that he unzipped himself and pulled down his jeans, revealing a growing bulge protruding through his jockey shorts.

I glanced down for a moment and took in the view, knowing that as I did so, it would get him harder. His hand ran slowly across his groin and then rested on his cock.

'Come on, touch it. You know you want to.' He ran his thumb along the outline of his erection and then cupped himself gently under his balls.

I looked back up at him and saw the wicked glint in his eye. It struck me how this would have driven me crazy just a few months ago – just seeing his desire for me would have made me want to jump on him and fuck him breathlessly.

Not any more. I watched this man sitting there, holding his stiff dick right in front of me, and knew that I didn't want *him* at all.

'I think you should put your trousers back on and behave – we're friends, let's keep it that way, OK?'

'You didn't used to say that, Abby, I know what you're like!' he said, as he grabbed my hand and attempted to place it onto his lap.

'Now, now, none of that!' I said, trying to be polite. 'I'd really prefer not to, if you don't mind.'

'Really?' He seemed disappointed. 'You not attracted to me any more, then?'

I tried to think of the most honest and least insulting way possible to let his ego down gently. 'Um, well, there's this guy and I really like him [*though he doesn't know it*], and although we're not "in" something [*but I wish we were*], I just want to see how things go and not shag anyone else right now [*because he means more to me than just sex*].'

He laughed. 'Ah, monogamy – that old game. You're a serious one, aren't you?' He seized my hand again and tried to get me to touch him once more.

I snapped my hand back. 'Yeah, I'm far more serious than you know, actually. It must be my degree in sarcasm that had you confused.'

'Quite likely, though I must say I am rather surprised, given our previous dalliances,' he replied, grinning. I noticed that his hand was slowly rubbing his cock through his underwear. I also noticed that I wasn't turned on at all.

'Look, I'll go make us tea, you put your clothes back on, and everything will be fine,' I tried to reason.

'With this?' he exclaimed, gesturing towards his now

rather pointed erection which was poking through his pants. 'I think this is going to have to get some air.'

And with that he pulled down his pants altogether.

I sat there and stared at him. He seemed rather pleased that his meat and two veg were on full display before me and reached down to grip himself.

'Touch it. Go on. Touch it. Please ...' he pleaded.

'No. I'm not going to. I don't want to,' I said. And as an afterthought, 'Sorry.'

That didn't stop him. His eyes were shining brightly as he watched me, his cock in his hand, slowly stroking it.

'OK then, you won't mind if I sort myself out, I've really got the fucking horn right now,' he said, rubbing his cock faster, the pre-come glistening on the head.

For a moment I thought about telling him to fuck off, that if he wanted a wank, he should at least go into the bathroom and do it privately, that I didn't want to have to witness him doing it, but given that just a few months ago, my mouth would have been wrapped around his cock, and my hand sliding in between my own legs, I felt bad that I was shutting him out so coldly. It seemed mean to be so harsh with him, under the circumstances.

Plus – and more importantly – he was fixing my ever-so-sick computer for free, so the least I could do was let him rub one out, as a way of saying thank you.

'Just don't get any of it near my laptop, OK?' I said, as I handed him some tissue, recalling that he fired off quite some distance when he came.

'Don't worry, I'm very neat, and I have good aim,' he said, somewhat unconvincingly.

I watched him as he got close, surprising myself when I

did not find it in the least bit erotic or arousing in any way – unusual for me, given that I have loved watching men masturbate before.

What I did find gripping – so to speak – was his expression. He watched me watching him, and his face turned from frustrated sexual need to one of rapturous delight; as he saw me smile whilst he ejaculated into his hand.

'Good boy,' I said, as he caught every last drop in the tissue.

'Right, that's better, I can concentrate now,' he said, pulling up his pants and trousers, 'and your computer looks like it's all good now, too.'

Eventually my computer got sorted, although I didn't, but this wasn't to my disappointment. On the contrary, I have learned that even when faced with a cock waved in front of me, I can turn it down, that there is more to life than revisiting sex with old fuck-buddies, and that in any situation you should always have tissues at the ready – you never know when they might come in handy. Literally.

Saturday 24th December

Although I tried to have no expectations about last night, I still got on the tube to meet Blog Boy filled with some hope, despite my insecurity, about how things stand. I couldn't help but want to have sex with him, not only because of our amazing chemistry, but because I have missed being intimate with him.

So I still shaved and trimmed all the necessaries, wore a new set of see-through black pants and bra, and rolled on some hold-up stockings. Presumptuous, I know, but there's a part of me – a stupid part, perhaps – that thought that maybe if he saw me like this, he might think me beautiful and that perhaps he would want me for more than just sex.

The evening went well. It was fabulous to see him again after several weeks of not hearing a word. Time went by so quickly that before I knew it, six hours had passed and we'd both missed our last trains. I was about to suggest that I called a mini-cab to take myself home, when he asked me if I would like to come back to his place. I was relieved. If we were going to be so intimate again, I wanted it to be him that initiated it, not me.

And he did.

We had beautiful sex. All night. We barely slept in between each session. His sex drive is just like mine – it's wonderful – he never tires of fucking, and he kept making me climax, like one long eternal orgasm. I just kept coming and coming. It was glorious.

But what was so special was the closeness between us; it seemed different, more intimate than before and there was one particular moment that was very intense for me. He was spooning me from behind and I had already climaxed, I don't know … five times already. I was close again and I turned my body so I could see his face. He was watching me and we both looked at each other intensely.

I suddenly felt more connected with him than I have ever been, as if in his expression, he was showing a depth of feeling for me that I hadn't seen before. I was overwhelmed with a sudden desire to tell him how much I felt for him and how this moment was about us being together, and not about the sex, that I didn't want it to end.

I wanted to tell him that I have finally realised that I want a relationship again, that my feelings for him have slowly developed over this year and about how I had tried to forget him when he had gone travelling, because I didn't want to be hurt. How I had fucked other men, not only because I wanted to have fun, but lately, so that I could get him out of my mind and move on, and how having sex with him again and again kept stirring up all those thoughts and feelings, making me realise just how strongly I felt.

But instead, in my insecurity, all I could do was run my fingers over his face and smile at him, hoping that through my touch, he would see how much he meant to me.

He smiled back at me as I stroked him and with that, I climaxed again and turned away from him, pulling him deeper into me as I felt his orgasm approach.

During the night he always sought out my feet with his and rested them against mine. A small gesture, but one that made me feel all the more close to him. With his arm around me as we slept, I wondered if perhaps he now saw me as some-one he could be in love with. I wrapped my arms around him too and felt that, at least for this night, I could pretend there was something more than sex between us.

But I know that I have to find out how he feels – all this sex with him is just distracting me from the inevitable. And it's making me hurt inside.

Monday 26th December

There's nothing like being cooped up indoors for a few days with all your relatives to get your blood boiling. And I don't mean boiling with fury here, though in my case, the level of frustration I feel has been pretty furious.

I am referring to my sexual frustration, which has been made all the more difficult to cope with due to the regular and close proximity of family members. Picture the scene –

INT. BEDROOM. MORNING
Me lying in bed, hand between my legs. My breathing is deep, my body moving slightly against my hand. The bed squeaks. I stop moving.

Cut to:

INT. KITCHEN. MORNING
My mother and father preparing breakfast.

Cut back to:

INT. BEDROOM. MORNING
My body moving back and forth. I slide my fingers between my legs, wetting them. I moan, then have to stop myself; trying to breathe silently through my nose. Suddenly:

MY MOTHER
Abby, are you awake?

My fingers stop moving. I lay there motionless.

ABBY
Uh, yeah …

MY MOTHER
Do you want some tea?

ABBY

Um, no thanks

I quickly resume fiddling, concentrating on keeping
the bed perfectly still. My fingers are slippery and
wet now. I slide two of them inside, gasping quietly
as they went in. I pretend they are Blog Boy's cock
inside me and I drift away into the fantasy, until:

MY MOTHER

Well, do you want some
coffee, then?

The cock disappears. I groan, stop moving my
fingers, and open my eyes.

ABBY

Yes, I'd love some, thanks.
Be down in a sec.

Silence; good. I close my eyes again, and think
about running my tongue around Blog Boy's chest,
stopping to kiss his nipples. I begin to throb
again, and resume my position, sliding my fingers
back inside. I can almost taste his skin …

MY MOTHER

Do you want cream or milk
with that? I know you like
cream; I made sure we got
enough, so would you like
that instead?

ABBY
(under my breath)
For fuck's sake
(raising my voice)
Yes, please, that'd be lovely

MY MOTHER
Well, are you coming down,
then?

ABBY
I'll be one sec

MY MOTHER
OK, it's on the table

ABBY
Thanks

I begin to rub myself frantically, whilst also trying to keep quiet and stop the bed moving. I was almost there, on the brink, when:

MY MOTHER
What are you doing up there?

I stop dead. What could I say? Guiltily, I move my fingers away.

```
                    ABBY

                  (urgently)

          I'm just in the middle of
          texting someone; gotta finish
          it off, won't be a minute


                  MY MOTHER

          Oh, OK, then. Don't blame me
          if it gets cold
```

I breathe a sigh of relief and refocus on my objective: an orgasm – and pronto. I thrust my fingers back down again, frig away silently and moments later, with a repressed shudder, an almost inaudible groan, and some mild teeth grinding, I finally climax.

When the last spasm wears off, I jump out of bed and grab a dressing gown. I pop to the loo, wash my hands and hop downstairs to join everyone else, hoping that no one notices the flush covering my face and neck.

It wasn't until I lift the (semi-cold, but very delicious) coffee to my lips that I became aware that the biggest give-away of all was still mildly perceptible: my fingers still smell of my pudenda.

I smile to myself. I got away with it – this time.

Thursday 29th December

I saw Blog Boy again last night. Unsurprisingly we ended up in bed together once more, pouncing on each other after a meal out. I tried not to shag him, I really did, but my desire was too strong. When his hand grazed my arse as we walked down the street, I felt myself respond inevitably and longed for more of his touch.

But when we got back to his place, I knew that I had to pluck up the courage to talk to him; I couldn't go into the New Year not knowing where things stand – it's doing my head in.

As if he knew what was on my mind he broached the subject first, just after we'd collapsed exhausted onto his bed from a wonderful long shag.

'So, have you had any Christmassy action?' he asked.

'What do you mean?' I replied.

'You know. Any other shagging?'

I was stunned that he had asked me that. Surely he knew that I only wanted to be with him now? Could he really think that I would want another man as well? 'No,' I said, quietly. 'You're the only person I have slept with recently.'

He was silent for a moment. 'Anyone you fancy then, that you want to snog?'

No, just you. I am falling for you and wish you were for me too. 'No,' I said, even more quietly. 'No one at all.' I paused. 'What about you?'

He shook his head, 'No'.

I wondered why he had asked me that. Perhaps he was just being my mate and making idle chit-chat. But maybe there was a possibility that he felt something more for me too and was testing the water to see how serious I was about him. I knew I had to tell him how I felt – it was now or never.

So I took a deep breath and asked him what he wanted from being with me.

Hesitating for a moment, he told me he was unsure, that

his gut instinct was that he didn't see anything happening with us – he couldn't see a future with me.

I felt myself go numb, as if I was observing the events from outside my own body. I nodded at him, an automatic response to the gnawing feeling that was slowly making its way from the pit of my stomach up to my heart.

Blog Boy took my hand, nervously smiled at me and then asked me what I wanted from him.

That was when I felt the tears well up in my eyes. I couldn't help it. 'I, um, I had hoped that we might get into something,' I said, trying not to look in his eyes, for fear that if I did, the tears would pour out of mine. 'I've started to realise that I care about you, that I want more than just being friends and this' – I gestured to our entwined bodies. 'But, er, I guess not …'

Blog Boy gripped my hand harder. 'Abby, I'm sorry. It's not that there isn't attraction between us – clearly there is – I like you *very* much; you are terrific company. But I just don't feel that *thing* … the chemistry … where you *know* you want to be in a relationship with somebody – it's not there for me. And I've considered it – I've thought about it, but it just hasn't happened for me. Sorry.'

I bit my lip, holding back the tears. They could come later – when I was alone. 'I understand,' I said, calmly, as if it were the most normal, relaxing thing in the world to be rejected by someone you cared deeply for. 'It's fine. I'll be fine.'

He smiled at me. 'And we'll still be friends – yeah?'

I nodded, whilst thinking – *but we can no longer be friends that fuck: I can't deal with that any more.*

We kissed and lay in each other's arms. As I drifted off to sleep, I felt a mixture of emotions: relief that I finally knew where things stood between us, frustration that I wouldn't be able to continue having fantastic sex with him, and sadness that he didn't want to be with me.

I know it's stupid, and I need to focus on positive things, but as I curled up with him next to me, I couldn't stop myself thinking, What's so wrong with me that he doesn't want to be with me?

Saturday 31st December

It's weird. The last few days I've felt oddly content. Mildly happy, even. I thought I would be more upset about Blog Boy, that I would be crying buckets of tears. After so long liking him it'd be normal to weep more than just a little when he rejected me, surely?

But I feel detached from it and calm, somehow. I don't feel overly emotional, just sad that things didn't work out. Maybe a part of me knew that it wasn't going to work out. Maybe I had been preparing for that all along.

What I do feel sad about, though, is this: tomorrow is a New Year and I am still single – and shagless – and I don't want to be.

Last year I lived my life as a single woman quite happily. I wasn't looking to get involved with a guy, I didn't want the hassle of dealing with their baggage. I think this was partly due to my feeling betrayed by Steven and then not trusting men as a result, but partly it was because I just wanted to have some laid-back fun with no strings attached.

And I have. Boy, I have. It's been a good time all round: I have enjoyed all my experiences, even the bad ones.

But the thing with Blog Boy threw me a little. There I was living it up as a single woman and yet in him I felt as though I had found something I wanted – something more than just one night of hot shagging.

I used to think that good orgasms were what was important and that if a guy was good in the sack I would be content.

Since the experiences I shared with Blog Boy I have come to the conclusion that even the best sex in the world can be unfulfilling in the long term. I need something more now. I may be a sex fiend, but even the thought of multiple orgasms with a fantastic lover has begun to feel empty to me, because there is no emotion involved in the process.

Over the last few days, I have discovered something else: maybe the reason I am not overwhelmed with sadness about it not working out with Blog Boy is that I wasn't actually in love with him. Perhaps, instead, I was in love with the *idea* of him. Maybe Blog Boy represented that which I didn't think I wanted until recently: a relationship. I do want a partner. I can now see that they might be a positive addition to my life, rather than a hindrance.

I am beginning to understand that I *am* just like any other girl: I too want someone to cuddle at night and who'll watch me fall asleep; someone who will know the real me; someone who wants to love me as well as make love with me. And maybe there are other women just like me too, girls with ravenous sex drives who want to shag all the time.

When I now see other women partnered up, with the babies, the career – it seems to me that they have it all, including the sex, and that although I feel happy and successful in my own life and love shagging with abandon, I am also lonely.

So maybe I do need the mental thing, the closeness, the

companionship and all that malarkey once again. Maybe I do need to be in *love* instead of in *lust*. Maybe I *want* to make love again too.

But sex is – and always will be – very important to me; I have been with partners where it was not a prority for them, and it left me very unhappy. So as a bare minimum, my part-ner would need to have a good libido and not be put off by mine being high.

Certainly, when faced with a man who says, 'I'm far too tired to shag, but why don't you play with yourself and tell me all about it in the morning, when you are riding my cock,' or a man who says, 'You're horny *again*? God, what are you, some kind of nymphomaniac?' and then turns away from me and goes to sleep, I would go with the former every time.

So with that in mind, sex *is* very important. Or rather, a man's *attitude* to sex is what is important and I think it is this that I am going to have to remember if I want to find that special someone.

Because although I now want more than just a shag from a bloke, I also know that it'll be a *special* kind of man who understands and appreciates that I'm a girl who wants to be thrown on the dining room table and fucked hard from behind when our kids are asleep.

I'm optimistic that such a man is out there. I hope to find him – and soon. It's time to settle down, I think. But I also plan on continuing to have fun while I'm out searching for him. After all, a girl's gotta shag a few frogs before she finds her prince, hasn't she?